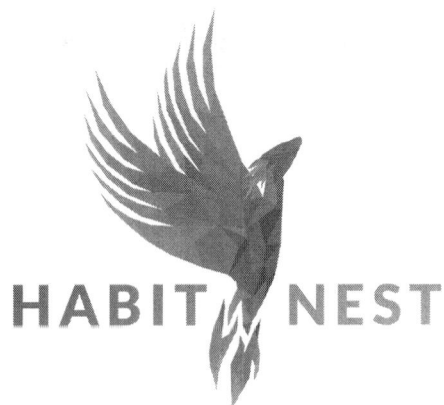

HABIT NEST

Your home for building healthy lifestyle habits.

HabitNest.com

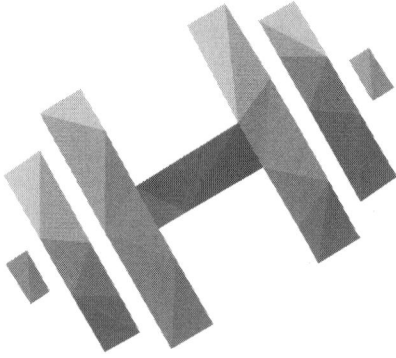

THE WEIGHTLIFTING
GYM BUDDY JOURNAL

Volume 1 of 3

Your pocket personal trainer.
Just get to the gym,
we'll do the rest.

Created with love by
Amir Atighehchi, Ari Banayan, & Mikey Ahdoot

Exercises Disclaimer:

The exercises provided by Habit Nest™ (and habitnest.com) are meant to serve as a general guide and are not to be interpreted as a recommendation for a specific treatment plan, product, or course of action. The exercises provided are not without their risks, and this or any other exercise program may result in injury. They include, but are not limited to: risk of injury, aggravation of a pre-existing condition, or adverse effect of over-exertion such as muscle strain, abnormal blood pressure, fainting, disorders of heartbeat, and very rare instances of heart attack. To reduce the risk of injury, before beginning this or any exercise program, please consult a healthcare provider for appropriate exercise prescription and safety precautions. While this is an exercise guide, it is not intended to be a direct fit for each person. It is imperative that each person tweaks the program to work for them in a way that suits their personal needs best, especially from a safety standpoint. Do not perform any exercises that cause you pain in any way. Consult with a certified personal trainer to help guide you through each exercise in person to assure they are all being done properly and in ways that will minimize injury.

The exercise instruction and advice presented are in no way intended as a substitute for medical consultation. Habit Nest™ disclaims any liability from and in connection with this program. As with any exercise program, if at any point during your workout you begin to feel faint, dizzy, or have physical discomfort, you should stop immediately and consult a physician.

Information Disclaimer:

The information provided by Habit Nest™ (and habitnest.com) is for educational and entertainment purposes only, and is not to be interpreted as a recommendation for a specific treatment plan, product, or course of action. Habit Nest™ does not provide specific medical advice, and is not engaged in providing medical services. Habit Nest™ does not replace consultation with a qualified health or medical professional who sees you in person, for the health and medical needs of yourself or a loved one. In addition, while Habit Nest™ frequently updates its contents, medical, health and fitness information changes rapidly, and therefore, some information may be out of date. Please see a physician or health professional immediately if you suspect you may be ill or injured. Before implementing any nutritional information provided, consult with a nutritionist as well to make sure you can fit your personal health and nutrition needs.

The Habit Nest Mission

We are a team of people **obsessed with taking ACTION** and **learning new things** as quickly as possible.

We love finding the **fastest, most effective ways** to build a new skill, then **systemizing that process for others.**

With building new habits, we empathize with others every step of the way *because we go through the same process ourselves.* We live and breathe everything in our company.

We use our hard-earned intuition to outline **beautifully designed, intuitive products** to help people live **happier, more fulfilled lives.**

Everything we create comes with a mix of **bite-sized information, strategy, and accountability.** This hands you a simple yet **drastically effective roadmap** to build **any skill** or habit with.

We take this a step further by diving into **published scientific studies,** the opinions of subject-matter **experts,** and the **feedback we get from customers** to further enhance all the products we create.

Ultimately, Habit Nest is a **practical, action-oriented startup** aimed at helping others take back decisional authority over every action they take. We're here to help people live **wholesome, rewarding lives** at the **brink of their potential!**

– Amir Atighehchi, Ari Banayan, & Mikey Ahdoot
Cofounders of Habit Nest

Table of Contents

***Note:** You'll also find content dispersed throughout the workouts to help improve your experience — things like Pro-Tips, Bonus Challenges, Common Form Issues, and more.*

205 Fin

214 Workout Index

Our Mission In Creating This Journal

Sometimes, it isn't easy to get to the gym.

Sometimes you're not sure what to do at the gym.

Sometimes when you get to the gym you don't feel like pushing yourself.

Sometimes, you need a Gym Buddy.

Our goal in creating this journal was to make it as easy as possible for you to get to the gym, have an amazing workout, watch incredibly fast progress happen right before your eyes, and ultimately feel supremely confident in your body.

We created this all in one personal trainer & tracker so that you don't have do ANY thinking when it comes to your workouts.

Having the journal removes any possible excuse for having an awesome workout, because the journal itself provides you with a way to be competitive with yourself so you can continue to see progress, without plateauing.

There is no guess-work. Your ONLY mission is to actually get in a gym and open the book. If you can make the commitment to get to the gym, open the book, and start the first exercise, you'll find yourself pushing harder than ever before without even realizing how it happened.

We created this journal to help you actually achieve your ultimate fitness goals.

The Key Factors of Weightlifting Success

How the Journal Works

Every day, you're going to be given a COMPLETE workout routine designating:

- Which muscles will be worked,
- Exactly which workouts to do (each will come with complete explanations, guiding images, and alternative exercises),
- How many sets (how many times you'll begin and end a complete round of an exercise) you'll do of each workout, and
- The rep range (the number of contractions) you're aiming for on each set.

You have two tasks to complete every day you choose to workout:

1. <u>Before you get to the gym (or right before you start)</u>: Look at what the day's workout consists of - which exercises you'll be doing - and read the explanations and images in the workout index in the back of the journal.

   To make it even easier, we included exercise guide links in the top left corner of each workout. These include the workout descriptions for that day as well as links to videos demonstrating how to perform them properly.

Until you're familiar with each exercise, it'll be annoying to keep looking back during your workout. It would be wise to get familiar with the exercises the night before or for a couple minutes before you begin.

2. <u>During your workout</u>: For each exercise, fill in the number of reps you complete and the amount of weight you use. This is the most adequate way to track your progress.

   We designate tracking lines for all of this, you just have to write down the numbers.

We'll be aiming to complete 3 sets per exercise. There are a series of ways to challenge yourself as you progress through the journal as well.

You can up the sets completed from 3 to 4 per exercise (we included tracking for this on each workout page).

You can also push yourself further by completing a 'dropset' on every last set of each workout.

*A **'dropset'** is where you complete one round of an exercise and immediately lower the weight to do one more round to exhaust the muscle even more.*

We recommend setting a long-term goal of eventually reaching 4 sets and a dropset for each exercise. This ensures the portion of the muscle being worked is exhausted in each individual exercise.

Why 'Pyramid' Sets?

A pyramid set means we'll be starting each exercise with a lower weight and higher rep range. We'll progressively be *increasing the weight* while *lowering the number of reps* as we move from set to set.

There are many benefits to pyramid sets. Possibly the biggest benefit is that there is essentially a built-in warm up on the first set that allows the muscle to prepare for heavier lifting.

The lower rep range sets also give you a taste of what you're capable of. The amount of discomfort you face in your last few sets shows you how far you've come along. When you can complete your last few sets with relative comfort and ease, you know it's time to move up in weight with all four sets!

Pyramid sets force you to really test the limits of the muscle being worked. This leads to a greater understanding of your progress.

Push & Pull Muscle Groups

The combination of muscles that will be worked on any given day will vary.

In general, we'll combine one 'push' muscle with one 'pull' muscle rather than the traditional method of using multiple 'pull' or 'push' muscles.

The 'push' muscles are those which require a pushing action from the body to complete a movement. The most simple example is a push-up or using the bench press. The 'pull' muscles are those that require a pulling motion - the back and biceps are examples of pull muscles.

The reason we'll regularly combine one 'push' and one 'pull' muscle in each day's workout is that we'll be getting more of the body involved on a regular basis.

Tracking Your Weightlifting Progress

Strength training is about using either physical weights or our body-weight to contract our muscles under tension to stimulate growth, strength, power, and endurance.

The factors that determine the quality of our body's reaction to the training we put it through are:

1. *Frequency*: How often we train
2. *Intensity*: How hard we train
3. *Time*: How long we train
4. *Type of exercise*: What we do when we train

All of this boils down to one very simple principle:

> *Our bodies change when we regularly push their current limits.*

> *The moment your level of intensity becomes 'normal' is the moment you stop changing.*

If you're currently working out one day per week, then increasing to 2 or 3 times a week will have a significant impact on your progress.

If you already work out 4-5 times a week, you have to find alternate ways to increase intensity and push the limit to continue changing at the rate you want.

Between the four factors above, you always have something available to use that can increase the intensity with which you face your body's progress.

If you can continuously reach the point where you're really pushing the boundary of what your body is capable of, you'll always be making strides towards your goals.

This journal will help you consistently find that boundary - it's up to you to push past it.

Resting Periods Between Sets

It is important to pay attention to how much rest you take in between sets.

You need to give your muscles enough time to be ready for the next set while making sure you're not wasting time and are working with *maximum intensity*.

You'll need to find the proper balance for yourself. Your resting periods will decrease the more experienced you become.

In general, 30 seconds - 90 seconds in between sets is a good bench mark. Anything under may be too short, and anything over is probably too long.

What's important is that you learn to recognize when you're wasting time out of laziness and to limit that as much as possible!

How Often Should I Exercise?

This is a common question that is situational based on what's realistic for each person.

The journal is undated and structured to be used by what works for you, your goals, and your schedule.

As a frame of reference:

- **Light**: Exercise 2 days a week.

- **Medium**: Exercise 4 days a week.

- **Hard**: Exercise 5-6 days a week.

If you're driven enough to achieve the best results, you should set a long-term goal of building up to 5-6 workouts a week.

Targeting Each Part of Every Muscle

The muscles we focus on in weight training are the *Chest, Back, Shoulders, Biceps, Triceps, Trapezius, Quadriceps, Hamstrings, Glutes, Calves, and Abdominal Muscles.*

Chest

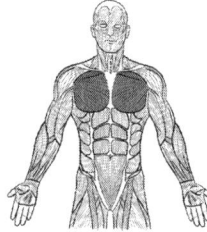

The chest (pectoral muscle) is one of the bigger muscles on the upper part of our body. As such, no one workout will adequately target the entire chest area.

Chest workouts will either *mainly* target the upper chest, middle part of the chest, or the lower chest. Focusing on all three major areas will allow the muscle to develop fully for maximum growth, thickness, and strength.

Back

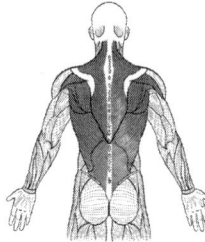

The back covers an enormous part of our upper body and, like the chest, will require many different types of exercises to ensure that each part is being targeted adequately.

Back workouts are generally split into those that target the latissimus dorsi ('lats' or 'wings'; the muscles behind your abdomen) and exercises that target the muscles closer to the top of our backs (the entire area in between our shoulder blades).

Shoulders

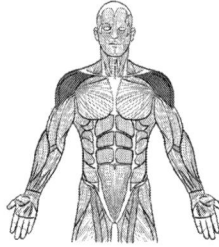

Shoulder development is crucially important in weightlifting, partially because shoulder development improves the way the biceps, triceps, chest, and back look.

More importantly, the shoulders are at work when performing most upper-body exercises and thus need to be strong enough to perform those exercises without risking injury.

Shoulder workouts generally work the entire muscle. However, the muscle is split into three distinct parts - front, medial, and lateral, which all require unique workouts to develop the muscle in its totality.

Biceps

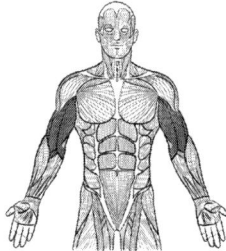

As one of the smaller muscles on our bodies, the biceps tire out more quickly than bigger muscles like the chest or back, and, due to muscle size, simply cannot grow as strong.

Bicep workouts will focus on making sure we hit the long-head and short-head of the muscle (inner and outer parts).

Triceps

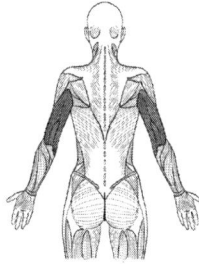

Tricep development is really important to arm strength and size because the tricep makes up more than 50% (around 2/3rds) of your arm. Triceps have 3 'heads' (hence the name) - lateral, medial and long. Most workouts hit all 3, but each requires unique attention, which we'll definitely give them!

Abs, Obliques & Core

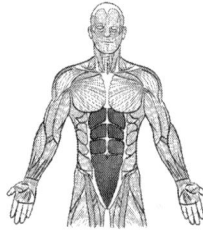

Your abdominal muscles consist of the rectus abdominis (six-pack), external obliques, and internal obliques. Abs are smaller muscles and require less training, but as smaller muscles, the recovery periods are also shorter - meaning you can train them more often.

The most important aspect in having visible abs is your body fat percentage, which is largely a result of the quality of your diet.

So we WILL train abs, but whether they show or not will be very dependent on how clean you eat.

Legs

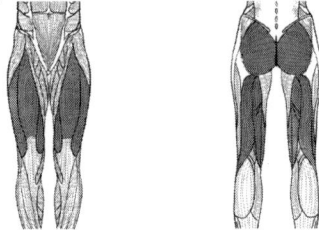

Our leg muscles are split into three general parts - quadriceps, hamstrings (and glutes), and calves.

We'll do bigger compound workouts that work the entire leg, but also do exercises to focus on each part of the leg individually.

Leg training is critically important because it boosts testosterone, allowing further growth of the rest of the body. Don't think when you're doing legs you're missing out on doing something that shows more.

Our lower bodies are a big part of how we look. They give the body the foundation it needs for healthy and active living and in fact allow the muscles on the upper body to grow.

Mind-Muscle Connection

"What puts you over the top? It is the mind that actually creates the body, it is the mind that really makes you work out.. it is the mind that visualizes what the body ought to look like as the finished product."
   - Arnold Schwarzenegger

The idea behind the mind-muscle connection is simple:

The more your mind is focused on the muscle being worked as it contracts, the greater your muscle development will be.

Acetylcholine is a neurotransmitter that stimulates your muscles to move.

The more you bring an active attention to the muscle being worked, the contraction in each and every rep, the more acetylcholine that's produced.

The more acetylcholine that's produced, the better the contraction, and the better the gains.

Therefore... **focused attention is very, very important.**

You can't study when your mind is wandering, right? You can't be productive when your thoughts aren't with what you're doing.

Working with the body in weightlifting is no different - active attention on what you're doing is essential.

Bring the importance of the mind-muscle connection to your attention at the very beginning of every workout and try to remember it throughout each set.

Become a Strategic Stretcher

Stretching is commonly done improperly (e.g. stretching muscles that are already overstretched) or is ignored altogether.

Instead of stretching random muscles, we recommend becoming a strategic stretcher. This means figuring out which of your muscles are tightest and have mobility issues, then stretching those specifically.

For example, if you have anterior pelvic tilt (a common issue, look it up if you're unfamiliar!), you would want to **stretch the following muscles:**

- Hip flexors
- Thoracic spine
- Lower back

And **avoid stretching:**

- Hamstrings

You'll also want to strengthen specific muscles that are weak and underused, leading to poor posture / mobility. In the example above, you'd want to strengthen your upper back (specifically the erector spinaei), your abs, and your glutes.

A fantastic resource for mobility exercises (and fitness in general) is the Athlean-X channel on YouTube. Jeff Cavaliere, the founder, has created many in-depth and science-based videos on improving mobility for specific body parts.

Paying Attention to the Inner & Outer Environment

Mindfulness is an important aspect of every workout. Not just for the mind-muscle connection, but also to understand your own internal limits of intensity, for safety, and respect.

Internally, what am I working with?

There's the struggle to reach my physical limit, which my psychological laziness can pull me from - where I know for a fact I'm not working hard enough because I'm wasting time, taking too long of breaks, etc. I need to constantly work against this.

There is also the internal consideration about what I look like. I have to keep in mind that how others are perceiving me is useless to the quality of my workout (unless it's positive because it helps me work even harder).

Everybody at the gym is there to do their own thing, worried about how they look. Worry about the workout, not what people are thinking about you!

Externally, I find myself in this place, a gym.

I'm not the only one here.

I need to understand that I am in relationship to this place, to the people here, to the equipment.

I need to bring an attitude of respect that will increase the quality of my workout.

I must carry with me a respect for the work I'm doing on my own body - not to waste the time I spend... A respect for the safety of my own body and the other people working out around me... A respect for the gym itself, for the staff, and for the equipment.

The main thing is, I have to constantly bring my attention back into the gym when my thoughts slip away.

Focusing and understanding what I'm doing will show me how to improve and increase the intensity of every workout.

The Extreme Importance of Form

Before beginning any exercise, you have to be absolutely sure that you adequately understand how to complete the exercise without getting injured.

We provide explanations of each exercise in the back of this journal, but if you're ever unclear, it only takes 30 seconds to look any exercise up online or ask somebody who works in the gym!

Our bodies are masters of compensation.

Where the body can cheat, it will.

There must be a conscious vigilance to retain proper form.

And let's be very clear: Form is **vitally** important.

Without proper form:

1. There is always a *risk of injury.*
2. You're most likely *missing the target muscle* because you're *compensating with body parts that don't need to be used.*

There is zero reason not to use proper form on any given exercise.

We will explain what proper form is in every exercise we provide in the journal, **but if you're ever unclear, PLEASE search online for a video that delves further into how to perform the workout properly until you're confident you can complete it without getting hurt.**

Check your ego at the door, and make sure you can complete each exercise with the **amount of weight** that will allow you to **retain the right form.**

Not completing a rep because you're exhausted and can't do it without breaking form is one thing - a beautiful thing.

Hurting yourself to complete a rep with muscles that aren't supposed to be involved is another thing - an ugly thing.

Do the beautiful thing.

Bonus tip: a commonly ignored yet incredibly useful strategy is to record yourself doing a specific exercise so you can actually SEE your form vs. tracking it mentally.

What's the Deal with Cardio?

Look, cardiovascular and aerobic exercise are always important - both for overall health as well as weight loss/muscle development.

Traditional aerobic exercise (static exercise like running on a treadmill, biking, or using the elliptical machine) is obviously great for health purposes, but it is not the optimal cardiovascular work for burning fat.

<u>HIIT Cardio</u>

To really derive the benefit of keeping healthy on the inside while burning the most fat, we recommend HIIT cardio 2-3 times a week.

It's all about short bursts of intensity rather than longer, static routines.

One day per week of this journal is dedicated to doing a cardio routine which is likely different from your ordinary idea of what cardio should be.

We'll give you a specific routine of bodyweight exercises that you'll perform (in order) with very short rest periods (or none at all).

It helps keep you engaged, works on muscle toning while getting your heart rate up, and makes cardio just a little bit easier to do with a smile on your face.

If you're vehemently opposed to doing cardio, an approach you can take is an experimental one - try doing minimal cardio for 2-3 weeks (just the days in the journal, nothing extra) and see what happens to your body fat % over time. If your nutrition + weightlifting intensity is spot-on, and you're not burning as much fat as you'd like, you can introduce additional cardio days then.

Alternatively, if you want to guarantee your results and get maximum effectiveness off the bat and not risk wasting any time, start with the above suggestion of 2-3 cardio days a week for 20 minutes a session. Add an additional day per week if you're not seeing great fat loss results.

Cardio is a key factor to deploy when your fat loss is stalling - use it strategically, wisely, and without complaints.

The Importance of Workout Intensity

The truth is you need to have a very high level of intensity when weightlifting to see real progress.

Remember, *intensity is what makes or breaks a workout,* every day.

However, this is a VERY easy point to misread and not understand properly. The level of intensity you should push yourself to build in your workouts looks like:

- *Walking in the gym with the mentality of giving your ALL to the workout, not wasting a second or moment there and moving with a fiery, powerful sense of direction.*

- *Having complete mental focus to perform your absolute best each day.*

- *Minimizing distractions like using your phone during rest periods.*

- *Tracking your rest periods and not letting them linger on past 45-120 seconds. This may mean starting a set when you feel too tired to do it at your best, but doing it anyways.*

- *Having pure mental focus on maintaining proper form and pushing your body to its limit with each set (without risking injury to yourself).*

- *Pushing yourself to set NEW limits by challenging yourself to do an extra rep when you feel completely dead after a set (again, while prioritizing staying safe and avoiding injury).*

- *Removing the fear of not hitting your desired rep range and feeling like a failure; knowing that your true goal is to give each set everything you've got and reach muscle failure.*

- *Not showing your body mercy if it feels tired / craves long rest periods. Force yourself to push through and you will feel more energized.*

If you feel it's naturally difficult to achieve all this, know that reaching the proper intensity in your workouts is absolutely a *trainable habit* within yourself. Make it a long-term goal to challenge yourself in the gym to reach it.

To help hold you accountable to increasing your intensity, we added a 'Workout Intensity' tracker at the end of each workout where you can record how intense your effort was each day as a numerical rating out of 10.

Adequate Recovery

Soreness is GOOD!

You WILL feel sore.

You WANT to feel sore - that's one way you know you're doing work.

As you progress through this journal, you will notice your stamina and workout capacity increasing.

But that being said, recovery is a necessity. Pushing yourself to the limit is also necessary.

How do I find the balance?

Recovery involves more than just letting your muscles rest - it involves letting your joints, connective tissues, and bones rest as well. There is lots more involved in any weight training exercise than just the muscle itself.

Think of it as the same reason we need to sleep every single day. Letting the body rest is enormously important.

The beautiful thing is that your body will tell you when it needs to rest!

Physical exhaustion as opposed to mental fatigue becomes very obvious when the body has surpassed a certain point that you'll recognize.

Of course, that means you have to really feel the exhaustion rather than use recovery as an excuse to not push yourself or even get to the gym.

A big part of what you gain by weight training regularly is becoming sincere with yourself about when you're making excuses vs. when you really need a rest.

Regardless of how many days a week you decide to work out (we recommend 4-6 to really push yourself), getting adequate sleep is crucial to allow for proper muscle gain. If you notice your muscle growth is lower than usual, take a look at your sleep and see if you are getting enough each night based on what your body requires. Oftentimes, 8+ hours a night is optimal for enough recovery and muscle growth.

Optimizing Every Aspect of Your Nutrition

A Short Note on the Importance of Eating
You Can't Lie to Your Body

Our bodies are machines. Machines have a few main characteristics:
1. They respond in a unique way to external stimuli.
2. They need fuel to function properly and efficiently.
3. Maintenance is required to prevent degeneration.
4. They have many component parts, each with a definite function or 'job.'
5. All the parts of a machine taken as a whole make up a unit that has one particular function in which every part plays a role.
6. They are predictable. They can be manipulated to achieve desired results.

Think about your car. You buy a car because you have a need for a method of transportation – a way to get around. The car serves this overall purpose of taking you from place to place.

But a car isn't merely a mobility device. It has many parts which each play a role in creating the possibility of being your modern day horse. In the ignition system alone there are spark plugs, ignition wire, coil and distributor that control the timing and flow of electricity to the engine's cylinders...

Every week or so, you need to get gas for the car, right? Every few months or year, your car needs to be serviced.

If you want your car to be louder or faster, what do you do? You get someone to alter the exhaust system, or you change parts to increase all around power and torque.

You have a result you want to achieve... *Simply alter the machine to fit your vision.*

But you can't lie to your car. You can't tell it that you're giving it oil and give it orange juice instead.

The beauty of the human body is that it is a wonderfully intricate machine that responds mechanically to the appearance of new external stimuli, and it can be manipulated to achieve desired results the same exact way you can change the way a computer or car operates.

You can force your body to burn excess fat it holds by monitoring your macronutrient intake and obtaining the proper balance of nutrients.

But you can't tell your body to respond differently than what you put in it. Remember every day, every meal, every moment: *You cannot lie to your body.*

What About Supplements?

The most important thing to realize about supplements is that they're supposed to *supplement*.

They are not necessary, and come secondary (nowhere near) the importance of training regularly with intensity and eating clean.

Supplements on their own will not change your body/do the work for you.

They can, however, help you meet your macronutrient goals, assist in muscle recovery, and help facilitate overall health, which leads to better workouts.

There is a lot of information on different types of supplements to assist in achieving your weightlifting goals.

The two we'd like to recommend are some form of protein powder and a multi-vitamin.

If you're trying to gain muscle mass, eating enough protein is really important, and because it can be difficult to eat as much as needed, protein powder lessens the load.

Multi-vitamins simply help ensure that you're getting the basic nutrients you need even if you're not eating them!

Caloric Deficit & Macronutrient Ratios

The following is assuming that your body composition goals are to:

1. Have minimal excess body fat, and
2. Maintain or increase your body's muscle

Depending on the body you want, a proper balance needs to be struck between minimizing body fat and maintaining or increasing muscle. The food we eat is the single most important factor in both decreasing body fat and improving muscle definition.

Fat Loss vs. Weight Loss

Most people don't even scratch the surface when it comes to understanding what it means to 'lose weight.' Weight loss can come in a few different ways.

The loss of weight that shows up on a scale can either be the result of fat loss, muscle loss, or water loss.

We all have this goal of getting to an ideal weight we think will make us happy with our physique. But the number on the scale should be the least of your worries. The goal is always to be as fit as possible, be as healthy as possible, and most importantly, to be genuinely happy with your body just as it is.

The goal is to selectively manipulate the body to burn as much fat as possible, while retaining all the muscle we have on our bodies.

An example of the distinction between fat loss and weight loss is the very well-known 'no-carb' diet - complete elimination of all carbs from one's diet.

If you've heard people saying they're on a 'low-carb' or 'no-carb' diet that is working extremely well for them and quickly, here's why:

Every stored carbohydrate in your body holds 2.7 grams of water. Eliminating or seriously depriving your body of carbohydrates means you're losing a lot of water weight, which is good if you're looking to just drop the number on the scale quickly, but doesn't make sense if you want to achieve long-term weight loss and prevent future weight-gain.

There will always be people who make it work with any diet, but drastically lowering carbs for years on end isn't realistic for most people.

Achieving a Caloric Deficit

Note: Before following any nutrition advice in this journal, we recommend reaching out to your doctor and/or nutritionist to get their thoughts. This is because different people have different needs and it's always a good idea to check yours.

It's simple.

Your body needs a certain amount of energy to function.

A *calorie* is a unit of energy – it is the energy value of food.

When your body uses more calories than it takes in, it is forced to turn to other places to supply and fulfill the energy requirements it isn't getting from the food you're eating.

But the body has a few options for where it can go to take the energy that it needs. It can either go to fat stores, muscle protein, or a combination of both.

Our goal in achieving fat loss is to cause the body to undergo this process of finding alternate energy supplies, while doing all that we can to force the use of fat as the primary energy source rather than muscle.

When there is a caloric deficit and the body is forced to turn to alternate sources of energy, it is imperative to ensure that muscle catabolism doesn't occur.

Muscle catabolism is the breakdown of muscle tissue to supply energy for the body that isn't coming from the food we're eating. This is one of the main reasons people aren't necessarily happy with their bodies when they completely cut their carbohydrate intake.

To put everything into perspective, the moment you have a caloric surplus (you eat more calories than you burn), extra calories are stored as fat for future energy use in the event that it becomes necessary.

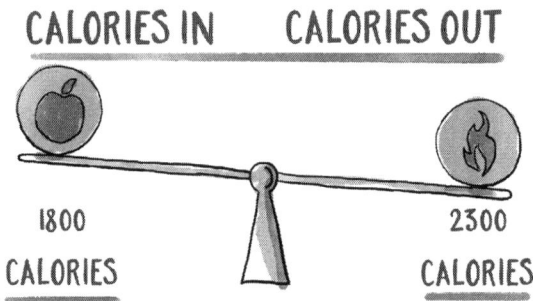

CALORIES IN   CALORIES OUT

1800 CALORIES   2300 CALORIES

Macronutrient Ratios

To lose weight, you need to eat less calories than you burn. But the name of the game when it comes to achieving FAT loss and preventing fat gain, is **understanding how the macronutrients you eat affect the body.**

Regardless of the extent of your caloric deficit, if your body isn't getting what it needs to function the way it was designed to operate, you will not be satisfied with the way you look. Instead, you will re-gain all the weight you lose the moment you start to eat like a human being.

The term **macronutrient** refers to the main types of food – carbohydrates, lipids (fats), and proteins.

The macronutrient ratio concerns the percentage of your caloric intake each of these three types of foods comprises.

To attain the right balance that will force your body to use fat for energy while retaining muscle, the macronutrient intake has to be carefully plotted and it must be tailored to your specific body type, the speed of your metabolism, and your ordinary activity levels.

Summary:

1. Your body needs energy to function, and is in a constant state of energy expenditure.
2. A calorie is a unit of stored energy; a measure of the value of food.
3. You can force your body to burn fat by achieving a caloric deficit.
4. A caloric deficit results where you burn more calories than you consume.
5. A caloric deficit may result in your body using muscle tissue for energy, which we can prevent with a proper balance of macronutrients.

Taking Action on Your Nutrition Goals

At this point, most people will take a mental note on these dietary / food points to apply going forward. But in order to **guarantee our results,** we must **guarantee we'll take action on this every day.**

As powerful as mindsets are, they are also very malleable and easily influenced by outside stimuli (like having a very common 'off day'). Meanwhile, systems (which provide accountability and tracking) are black and white - yes or no - 1 or 0.

We highly recommend putting together a structure you think can work in helping you stay consistent with your eating goals. Nothing is more demoralizing than aiming to feel better about yourself, working out hard for it, and seeing poor results (that you later justify).

After getting some clarity on which eating plan you want to follow (e.g. counting calories/macros or choosing a specific diet), there are a few ways to put it into effect.

As a free option

You can use a dietary tracking app, google sheet, or notepad to track calories/macros/ meals. Alternatively, you can use an extra whiteboard or calendar to track whether or not you hit your goals every day. If you think you can genuinely stay consistent with this for months / the long term, this is a great option.

As a paid option

We wrote *The Nutrition Sidekick Journal* for this exact reason - to provide a clear, unbreakable system to track your results and help you learn how to improve (without judgement!) at the same time.

If a pure tracking sheet is a bit too dull, redundant, and isn't stimulating enough for you, this may be the right choice.

Some things covered inside the *Nutrition Sidekick Journal*:

1. How to manipulate your body to burn fat while maintaining muscle
2. Tracking for your calories, water intake, and planned meals vs. actual eaten meals
3. New golden nuggets of information, pro-tips, daily challenges, and more each day

You can check it out at **habitnest.com/nutrition** and use discount code **TeamLean15** for 15% off if you decide to order one.

Effectively Tracking Your Progress

Tracking your progress is extremely important. That being said, the accuracy of your tracking is **even more important**. With flawed data that isn't actionable, your tracking is just an arbitrary, confusing, and often misleading number.

This section assumes you have two body-composition goals, which tend to be the most popular amongst people (and can be the healthiest):

1. You want to increase your muscle mass
2. You want to reach & maintain your body fat percentage at 8-15% (males) or 13-20% (females)

The problem with the scale

With weight training and fat loss, the scale's results (without deeper insight on it) can be your biggest enemy. This is because our shifts in bodyweight are affected by SO many factors, it's impossible to identify what has changed week by week with only a weight amount.

This is where **body fat tracking** comes in, right alongside **body weight tracking**. By combining the tracking of BOTH your body fat AND the scale, you're able to see exactly HOW your weight changed from week to week - whether you gained muscle, gained body fat, lost muscle, or lost body fat.

Accurately measuring your body fat percentage

There are many ways to do this, but the most cost-effective and practical way is to use a self-testing skinfold caliper. The one we recommend is the Accu-Measure as it costs roughly $10 on Amazon and has an existing scientific study backing up its effectiveness (it's within 1.1% accuracy of using an underwater body fat measurement, which is one of the highest levels of accuracy we have for measuring body fat).

Disclaimer: We have no affiliation with the Accu-Measure and aren't getting paid in any way for this recommendation. It's simply a great tool.

With the upsides being ease of use and cost, the biggest downsides of this method are the **potential inaccuracy** if you don't know how to measure yourself properly each week. Although it's **very possible to be incredibly accurate** with this method… it takes a good deal of practice. Thankfully, the product comes with step-by-step guide that lays out how to use it as accurately as possible.

As long as you are measuring yourself in the same location weekly, even if your placement isn't perfect, you'll be able to have comparable results you trust week after week. Make your main goal in measuring be *consistency in measuring.*

How do I get the right data?

We recommend measuring yourself weekly for both body weight (with a scale) and body fat (with the Accu-Measure).

We want to eliminate as many factors that can cause data inconsistencies as possible. When taking your measurements, do it:

- At the same time of day (ideally mornings)
- With the same food/water intake that day (ideally none, do it right as you wake up)
- With the same amount of clothes on, and
- Without holding any objects that could throw your readings off (e.g. your phone)

You can write this data down as you progress through the journal (in the next section) or record it on a note on your phone. If you choose the latter, make sure you don't hold your phone as you're measuring yourself.

Common misunderstandings with the Accu-Measure

After using the Accu-Measure ourselves, a few things were a bit unclear from the instruction sheet they provided. We spoke with a rep on the phone who helped clarify these points for us:

1. Where is the iliac crest?
To find your iliac crest, it should be near your waist line (like where you wear a belt) and you feel a big bone protruding out, towards the side of your body.

2. How can you measure consistently and accurately?
If you place the caliper directly on your skin, the ends will measure 2.5 inches exactly. You can use this to consistently grab the same distance each measurement.

Once you have grabbed your skin fold with your thumb and index finger, position the caliper halfway between the back of your skinfold (point closest to your body) and the front of the skinfold (point furthest from your body), 1cm away from your fingers.

Getting even more clarity, reducing measuring inaccuracy

The most important thing with using the Accu-Measure is **measuring yourself the same way week-to-week**. Even if you're measuring yourself improperly, or the Accu-Measure itself is inaccurate, your **week-to-week changes should remain consistent** as the method of measuring is consistent.

If you want to take this to the next level, or see how close to accurate your Accu-Measure is, you can get a detailed body scan (e.g. a water displacement scan) and see how it compares to the Accu-Measure. If a discrepancy exists, you'll at least know by how much and be able to mentally keep that in mind.

Write down the following each week:

1. *Measure your **total body weight** using a scale*

2. *Measure your **body fat %** using an Accu-Measure*

3. *Take your total body weight (#1) in pounds and multiply it by your body fat % (#2). This will give you your **body fat weight**.*

4. *Take your **total body weight** (#1) and subtract your **body fat weight** (#3) to get your **lean body mass**.*

Your lean body mass consists of every part of your body that's not considered fat (muscles, tissues, bones, organs, water weight, etc.) Since a significant changing factor in weight of your lean body mass is your muscle mass, we can use lean body mass as a near-accurate measure of fluctuations in muscle gain / loss.

The biggest inconsistency with your lean body mass will be the fluctuations in your water weight. Be mindful of this and how certain factors (e.g. being dehydrated, drinking lots of water, intaking too much sodium the day before) can affect this. If something seems wrong, give it at least 2 weeks before jumping to conclusions of whether your plan is or is not working.

What should I do with this measurement data?

The next two pages provide a space to record this data weekly over a 12 week period, followed by actions steps for how to adjust weekly for each scenario. Having this data recorded next to each other will allow you to spot trends in your weekly fluctuations and make the correct adjustments of action steps based on this.

Adjusting Based On Your Progress

As recommended in Tom Venuto's *Burn the Fat, Feed the Muscle*, you should make the following tweaks based on your weekly fluctuations of **body fat weight (B.F. Weight)** and **lean body mass (L.B.M.)** to achieve body fat loss & muscle gain:

1.   *If:* | B.F. Weight (↑) | | L.B.M. (↑) |

Then: Decrease your caloric intake (recommended: 100-200) and increase your cardio.

2.   *If:* | B.F. Weight (↓) | | L.B.M. (↑) |

Then: This is the holy grail and we are all jealous of you. Keep doing what you're doing. This is decently rare to occur, so treat it as a huge gift if you're experiencing it!

3.   *If:* | B.F. Weight (↑) | | L.B.M. (↓) |

Then: This is unlikely and usually due to a measurement inaccuracy. Alternatively, this may be due to factors outside of your training and nutrition, such as being under a lot of stress and not getting adequate rest. Recheck your results, and if they're accurate, take care of yourself and see if you notice a significant difference the following week.

4.   *If:* | B.F. Weight (↓) | | L.B.M. (↓) |

Then: Eat more calories (recommended: 100-200) and increase protein intake if you're under 1g * your total body weight.
Increasing your weight training intensity will help here as well.

5.   *If:* | B.F. Weight (↑) | | L.B.M. (—) | (This '—' icon means "stayed the same.")

Then: Eat less calories (recommended: 100-200) and slightly increase your cardio.
Note: This action step also applies if both your L.B.M. and your body fat weight stay the same (no change as the week before).

6.   *If:* | B.F. Weight (↓) | | L.B.M. (—) |

Then: This is fantastic! You're right on track, keep doing what you're doing.

Weekly Progress Tracker

WEEK 1

DATE: _____

WEIGHT: _____ BODY FAT %: _____

FAT WEIGHT: _____ LEAN BODY MASS: _____

ADJUSTMENTS TO MAKE

	{CIRCLE}			(FILL IN AMOUNT)
CALORIES	↑	↓	—	_____
CARDIO	↑	↓	—	_____
TRAINING INTENSITY	↑	↓	—	

WEEK 2

DATE: _____

WEIGHT: _____ BODY FAT %: _____

FAT WEIGHT: _____ LEAN BODY MASS: _____

ADJUSTMENTS TO MAKE

	{CIRCLE}			(FILL IN AMOUNT)
CALORIES	↑	↓	—	_____
CARDIO	↑	↓	—	_____
TRAINING INTENSITY	↑	↓	—	

WEEK 3

DATE: _____

WEIGHT: _____ BODY FAT %: _____

FAT WEIGHT: _____ LEAN BODY MASS: _____

ADJUSTMENTS TO MAKE

	{CIRCLE}			(FILL IN AMOUNT)
CALORIES	↑	↓	—	_____
CARDIO	↑	↓	—	_____
TRAINING INTENSITY	↑	↓	—	

WEEK 4

DATE: _____

WEIGHT: _____ BODY FAT %: _____

FAT WEIGHT: _____ LEAN BODY MASS: _____

ADJUSTMENTS TO MAKE

	{CIRCLE}			(FILL IN AMOUNT)
CALORIES	↑	↓	—	_____
CARDIO	↑	↓	—	_____
TRAINING INTENSITY	↑	↓	—	

WEEK 5

DATE: _____

WEIGHT: _____ BODY FAT %: _____

FAT WEIGHT: _____ LEAN BODY MASS: _____

ADJUSTMENTS TO MAKE

	{CIRCLE}			(FILL IN AMOUNT)
CALORIES	↑	↓	—	_____
CARDIO	↑	↓	—	_____
TRAINING INTENSITY	↑	↓	—	

WEEK 6

DATE: _____

WEIGHT: _____ BODY FAT %: _____

FAT WEIGHT: _____ LEAN BODY MASS: _____

ADJUSTMENTS TO MAKE

	{CIRCLE}			(FILL IN AMOUNT)
CALORIES	↑	↓	—	_____
CARDIO	↑	↓	—	_____
TRAINING INTENSITY	↑	↓	—	

WEEK 7

DATE: _____

WEIGHT: _____   BODY FAT %: _____

FAT WEIGHT: _____   LEAN BODY MASS: _____

ADJUSTMENTS TO MAKE
(CIRCLE)   (FILL IN AMOUNT)

CALORIES   ↑   ↓   —   _____

CARDIO   ↑   ↓   —   _____

TRAINING INTENSITY ↑   ↓   —

WEEK 8

DATE: _____

WEIGHT: _____   BODY FAT %: _____

FAT WEIGHT: _____   LEAN BODY MASS: _____

ADJUSTMENTS TO MAKE
(CIRCLE)   (FILL IN AMOUNT)

CALORIES   ↑   ↓   —   _____

CARDIO   ↑   ↓   —   _____

TRAINING INTENSITY ↑   ↓   —

WEEK 9

DATE: _____

WEIGHT: _____   BODY FAT %: _____

FAT WEIGHT: _____   LEAN BODY MASS: _____

ADJUSTMENTS TO MAKE
(CIRCLE)   (FILL IN AMOUNT)

CALORIES   ↑   ↓   —   _____

CARDIO   ↑   ↓   —   _____

TRAINING INTENSITY ↑   ↓   —

WEEK 10

DATE: _____

WEIGHT: _____   BODY FAT %: _____

FAT WEIGHT: _____   LEAN BODY MASS: _____

ADJUSTMENTS TO MAKE
(CIRCLE)   (FILL IN AMOUNT)

CALORIES   ↑   ↓   —   _____

CARDIO   ↑   ↓   —   _____

TRAINING INTENSITY ↑   ↓   —

WEEK 11

DATE: _____

WEIGHT: _____   BODY FAT %: _____

FAT WEIGHT: _____   LEAN BODY MASS: _____

ADJUSTMENTS TO MAKE
(CIRCLE)   (FILL IN AMOUNT)

CALORIES   ↑   ↓   —   _____

CARDIO   ↑   ↓   —   _____

TRAINING INTENSITY ↑   ↓   —

WEEK 12

DATE: _____

WEIGHT: _____   BODY FAT %: _____

FAT WEIGHT: _____   LEAN BODY MASS: _____

ADJUSTMENTS TO MAKE
(CIRCLE)   (FILL IN AMOUNT)

CALORIES   ↑   ↓   —   _____

CARDIO   ↑   ↓   —   _____

TRAINING INTENSITY ↑   ↓   —

Getting Started

Sample Workout: Biceps & Triceps

DATE _____

1. PREACHER CURL
(ALTERNATIVE: SEATED DUMBBELL CURL)

(Alternative exercises are listed here in case you can't properly do the given one. Always feel free to cross out any exercise and write your own!)

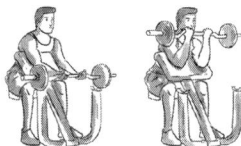

	PREVIOUS BEST	REPS: 5		WEIGHT: 60
SET 1		REPS: 14	(GOAL: 10-15)	WEIGHT: 40
SET 2		REPS: 10	(GOAL: 8-12)	WEIGHT: 50
SET 3		REPS: 7	(GOAL: 6-8)	WEIGHT: 60
SET 4 [OPTIONAL]		REPS: 6	(GOAL: 4-6)	WEIGHT: 60

(By having your 'Previous Best' reps and weight values listed for each specific exercise, you'll have a clear target to beat weekly.)

2. ZOTTMAN CURL

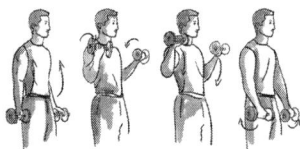

	PREVIOUS BEST	REPS: 6		WEIGHT: 20
SET 1		REPS: 15	(GOAL: 10-15)	WEIGHT: 15
SET 2		REPS: 12	(GOAL: 8-12)	WEIGHT: 17.5
SET 3		REPS: 8	(GOAL: 6-8)	WEIGHT: 20
SET 4 [OPTIONAL]		REPS: —	(GOAL: 4-6)	WEIGHT: —

3. ROPE HAMMER CURL

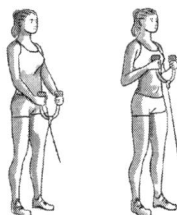

(The goal is to progressively increase weight on each set. Challenge yourself on EVERY set!)

	PREVIOUS BEST	REPS: 5		WEIGHT: 40
SET 1		REPS: 13	(GOAL: 10-15)	WEIGHT: 35
SET 2		REPS: 11	(GOAL: 8-12)	WEIGHT: 40
SET 3		REPS: 7	(GOAL: 6-8)	WEIGHT: 45
SET 4 [OPTIONAL]		REPS: 6	(GOAL: 4-6)	WEIGHT: 45

(Ideally, every set should be done to failure. The suggested ranges are meant to give you an aim for an adequate weight that will lead to failure within it.)

4. CONCENTRATION CURL

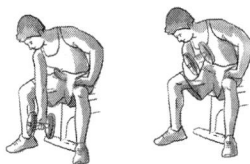

	PREVIOUS BEST	REPS: 4		WEIGHT: 20
SET 1		REPS: 14	(GOAL: 10-15)	WEIGHT: 17.5
SET 2		REPS: 12	(GOAL: 8-12)	WEIGHT: 17.5
SET 3		REPS: 8	(GOAL: 6-8)	WEIGHT: 20
SET 4 [OPTIONAL]		REPS: 6	(GOAL: 4-6)	WEIGHT: 20

AMOUNT OF CARDIO DONE TODAY:
20 min

34

Sample Workout: Biceps & Triceps

1. SKULL CRUSHER

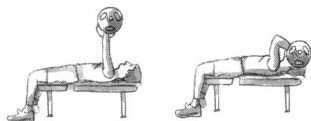

PREVIOUS BEST	REPS: 6		WEIGHT: 50
SET 1	REPS: 15	(GOAL: 10-15)	WEIGHT: 40
SET 2	REPS: 11	(GOAL: 8-12)	WEIGHT: 50
SET 3	REPS: 8	(GOAL: 6-8)	WEIGHT: 60
SET 4 [OPTIONAL]	REPS: 6	(GOAL: 4-6)	WEIGHT: 60

(The fourth set on each exercise is optional but highly recommended.)

2. CLOSE GRIP BENCH PRESS

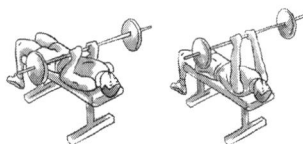

PREVIOUS BEST	REPS: 5		WEIGHT: 60
SET 1	REPS: 14	(GOAL: 10-15)	WEIGHT: 40
SET 2	REPS: 10	(GOAL: 8-12)	WEIGHT: 50
SET 3	REPS: 7	(GOAL: 6-8)	WEIGHT: 60
SET 4 [OPTIONAL]	REPS: —	(GOAL: 4-6)	WEIGHT: —

3. ROPE PULLDOWN

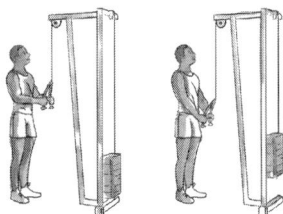

PREVIOUS BEST	REPS: 5		WEIGHT: 40
SET 1	REPS: 13	(GOAL: 10-15)	WEIGHT: 35
SET 2	REPS: 12	(GOAL: 8-12)	WEIGHT: 35
SET 3	REPS: 6	(GOAL: 6-8)	WEIGHT: 40
SET 4 [OPTIONAL]	REPS: 5	(GOAL: 4-6)	WEIGHT: 45

(Greyed sections are optional or won't apply to everybody! For example, here you'd fill it in if you were adding weights with a belt or using a seated/assisted dip machine.)

4. DIP
(ALTERNATIVE: ASSISTED DIP OR SEATED DIP W/ MACHINE)

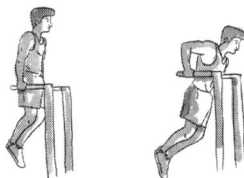

PREVIOUS BEST	REPS: 6		WEIGHT: —
SET 1	REPS: 7	(GOAL: TO FAILURE)	WEIGHT: —
SET 2	REPS: 7	(GOAL: TO FAILURE)	WEIGHT: —
SET 3	REPS: 7	(GOAL: TO FAILURE)	WEIGHT: —
SET 4 [OPTIONAL]	REPS: 6	(GOAL: TO FAILURE)	WEIGHT: —

TODAY'S WORKOUT INTENSITY:
8.5 / 10

The Three Factors of Behavior Change

James Clear, author of *Atomic Habits*, writes that there are essentially three parts to behavior change (we love your work, James!).

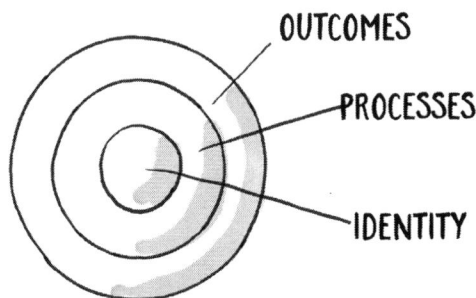

1. The Outcomes

The first is the outside layer: The Outcomes. This is synonymous with your goals (e.g. I want to achieve 15% body fat and have visible abs).

Outcomes are most useful at setting a larger, over-arching vision for where you want to go. The downsides of over-focusing on your outcomes are relying on hitting your goals to bring you happiness instead of enjoying the process, and a lack of practicality for what to do day-to-day.

Your outcomes are likely to change over the course of your life to match your ever-evolving goals and needs.

2. The Processes

The second, middle layer, is about processes — this boils down to what system and action steps you put in place to allow your outcomes to come to fruition. These are things like *I will go to the gym 4 times a week/ I will try to increase the reps and/or the weight of an exercise each time.* Processes are synonymous with strategies and tactics.

These can be very useful, especially when you find one that clicks, and you'll see a number for you to experiment with sprinkled throughout the journal.

These processes are likely to change over time as you test them out. See what works best for you and switch things up when you get bored / desensitized to them.

3a. Your Identity

This one's the big kahuna. This is the inner-most layer, matching who your internal belief is of yourself as a person. The biggest mistake people make in enacting behavior change is placing way too large of a focus on the first two parts of this puzzle, while entirely forgetting about the third and the most impactful — how you view yourself.

By properly emphasizing WHO you want to grow into, you will maximize your self-respect, satisfaction, and ability to control your actions — more than any motivation or strategy can give you. Your identity is what you can always fall back on to set your intuition, to guide you to what you should really be doing.

An example of setting your identity is:

"I'm someone who does what it takes to get lean, fit, strong, and healthy. I do what's right, not what's easy, in going to the gym and staying consistent with my nutrition and fitness goals."

*After defining the identity you want to grow into for yourself, chances are this will **not change much**, but rather, only **strengthen over time** based on your actions.*

3b. Your Identity On Your Off-Days

As much as this plays a role in building towards your goals, it's equally as important in regards to times where you fall off the wagon.

Most people subconsciously forget about what their self-identity looks like when this happens, allowing a massive negative self-view to kick in.

This leads to a major emotional factor, *guilt*, to kick in, and as many studies have shown, **guilt is a willpower destroyer** (these are cited at the end of the book).

Instead, mindfully set your identity in these situations…

Grow into the person who uses every opportunity of falling off-track to further strengthen your ability to *switch from your off-days back to being on-track.*

Chances are you won't have perfect consistency with your nutrition and fitness every single day, for the rest of your life, right? Life is about knowing which habits to employ, at the right time, to help you get the most fulfillment out of life.

This involves testing different things and seeing how they serve your life's purpose. In order to really do this, you must master the ability to switch back and forth and discover how to quickly rebuild the momentum you had with your habits, without any guilt that you "lost your mojo."

Be the type of person who can forgive yourself for your mistakes, who will love yourself unconditionally, and be a true best friend to yourself (because if you can't, who will?).

We know these are big emphases on emotional states that can come off as "fluffy," but the truth is our fulfillment in life is directly tied to our emotional states. Learning how to master them is the true feat of this journal, not just building up a specific habit.

Establishing Your Identity

Write your identity statements below.

What kind of person do you want to grow into through this process?

_____

_____

_____

_____

What kind of person do you want to be when you fall off the wagon of your habits? What do you want to remember about who you are and how you can repurpose these days to serve your life?

_____

_____

_____

_____

Common Weightlifting Myths

You can't build muscle and burn fat at the same time

Having experienced muscle gain alongside fat loss ourselves, we're happy to say this is false. Look, to build muscle your body has to have energy - we get energy through food. To lose fat, you have to burn energy. When you eat more than you burn, your body stores energy. When you burn more than you eat, your body loses energy.

The point is that your body uses existing fat for energy when you're at a caloric deficit. The energy is there and as long as you're eating enough of the right kinds of protein and carbs, you're protecting your body from burning through muscle as an energy source.

Another point to keep in mind is that although it is possible to have both muscle growth and fat loss occur at the same time, we recommend getting as lean as you'd like FIRST. This can be done via a 10-20% caloric deficit. Afterwards, you can prioritize muscle growth with a slight caloric surplus of roughly 10-20%.

The fastest way to lose fat is cardio.

Easily false. Your diet is the fastest way to lose weight, bar none. Even more importantly, although weightlifting loses the battle for weight loss against cardio when comparing them minute for minute, weight training will help burn more FAT. The number on the scale is one thing, but the way you look changes most based on the development of two factors - muscle development and lower body fat.

Your genetics determine everything.

Definitely not - it's the worst excuse for working on your body and it doesn't make any sense. Of course your bone length, the shape of your body, etc., all play a role in what you CAN look like at your maximum potential. But you can push your body to limits you never thought possible with weight training - you can completely transform the image you have of yourself in your head and in the mirror right now. You can get the body you want, no matter what shape and size you are right now.

Women bulk up when they lift weights.

It is REALLY hard to get big. To really grow and look the way you want, you have to work very, very hard. You have to want it for a very long time and work consistently towards it constantly refining as you go through the process. So no, picking up weights a couple times a week to have adequate, healthy muscle development will not make anybody grow big and bulky.

Falling in LOVE with the Process

There is no absolute correct way to work out.

The true secret to strength, muscle growth, and fitness is: you start SOMEWHERE with SOME routine, you stick to it for some time, learn from the experience and move forward from there.

We are giving you a routine that WILL 100% help change your body if you stick to it. But the learning never stops.

We hope this gives you the proper baseline to continue advancing in your weightlifting goals and strategies so you KEEP getting closer to that dream body.

This whole process is going to be a blast - seriously.

Whether you're experienced in weight training or just starting out, we promise, we will help push your boundary constantly. That's what we really fall in love with.

You'll learn about your own psychology...refine your body...grow in strength, size, endurance, and most importantly, you'll feel REALLY good.

You'll find that you regularly just have more energy. You'll consistently get a high from your workouts and you will begin to fall in love with the body in a special way.

The body is our home, the vehicle through which we travel this journey of life. It is infinitely complicated, wonderfully responsive, sensitive, and a primary instrument for inner psychological growth.

Keeping your body in order, inside and out, feels good for a reason.

That good feeling is how you know its importance - almost like how feeling hungry is your signal to eat.

Let's get to it!

Before Starting: Important Things to Keep in Mind for Each Muscle

Back

- Think of your hands as hooks - it's all about pulling. Your hands grip on and your back / lats should be doing all the work to move the weight.

- When you pull, actively push your chest out and elbows back, allows more of an extension a little more easily.

- Keep your back comfortably straight no matter which workout you're doing. Pulling and winging your back allows you to lift more weight at the expense of form and the best contraction of the muscle you're targeting. You want to avoid this as the contractions are what's important. Proper form leads to the best ones.

Biceps

- Similar to the triceps, keep your wrists straight as if a rod were going from your forearm through your wrist. Don't bend your wrist to ensure that the bicep is the part of the body making the movement.

- Keep your back flat. Maintain a neutral spine position without arcing forwards or backwards.

- Keep your elbows tucked into the body. They should remain still so that your bicep bears the burden of the movement and you're not getting help from the momentum of the rest of the body.

- Remember, the tension is desirable. The **contraction** is what we want - not just swinging around.

- If you feel you need to lift your elbow upward to finish the movement, your supporting muscles in your forearm are likely too weak - focus on your mind-muscle connection with them.

Chest

- Keep your chest out, traps back, and shoulders down.

Legs

- Number one rule - DO NOT SKIP!

- Whenever you train your legs there will be an increase in your body's testosterone. The more intense your workout is, the more testosterone that's produced. Leg training includes many exercises that work the entire lower portion of the body. As big movements that work many muscles at once, the intensity is very high, producing more testosterone, which benefits all of your growth - upper AND lower body.

Shoulders

- There is a lot of natural swinging that happens when we work shoulders. You have to stay mindful of that and not use momentum for the movement. The whole point is to maximize the muscle contraction, so using the momentum of the swing doesn't do much to help here. Doing 6 good reps is better than 15-20 swinging reps!

- Relax your shoulders and traps, let them fall *down* and *back*... and keep them there!

Triceps

- Keep your wrists STRAIGHT as if a rod were going through your forearm and hand. Don't let your wrist lag back or hold it too tightly forward.

- Keep your elbows tucked inwards to your body to contract as much of the tricep as possible and also hit the lateral head of the tricep.

- Keep your elbows in the same spot as you complete each movement. When your elbows moves up and down with the movement, you're compensating with the rest of your upper body and your tricep isn't bearing the entire load.

Note: You will see additional notes & illustrations about improving your form throughout the journal!

General Safety Tips

1. You always want the muscle you're working on to take the load, not your back or other parts of the body - all it takes is ONE bad set, ONE bad rep to set you back weeks or even months.

2. Never invent new uses for a machine!

3. When picking up weights, use proper form. Bend with your knees and use leg strength to pick up the weight. Doing so avoids injury from straining back and hips.

4. If you're unsure of whether you can complete a rep for a workout where you can't just drop the weights, USE a *spotter* - someone to help you finish the movement if you get stuck.

5. Don't extend to the absolute limit of your flexibility unless you're extremely comfortable with the exercise.

6. Don't just drop weights, they fall hard and bounce around. You can hurt others or yourself when you drop the weights from your hands to the floor. Use a controlled movement to place weights on the ground or in their proper place.

7. Fingers and toes are weirdly susceptible to getting hurt when picking up or putting weights down - watch out for it. Our cofounder Ari once bruised his finger because he put the weight on the rack too quickly and the dumbbell went over the rack with his finger caught in between it and the rack.

8. If you've made the very normal mistake of using a weight that's too heavy for you and you realize you need help because you're in a situation in which you're not sure what to do - ASK for help from somebody nearby!! *Side Story*: Ari was once a bit overzealous in benching - he couldn't complete a set and had to rest the bar on his chest, roll it to his hips, take off one plate from one side of the barbell. The imbalance of weight caused the bar to sway to one side (all the weights fell off) and then immediately to the other side (and all the weights fell off that side). It was EXTREMELY dangerous and he's lucky he didn't hurt himself or anyone else.. because he was too stubborn to ask someone for help.

9. Always be aware of your surroundings - make sure what you're doing doesn't jeopardize anybody else's safety.

10. Always lean on the side of safety rather than one of ego and lifting heavy or forcing yourself to break personal records. Most importantly, don't do anything that risks injuring yourself, which will set back your progress by a very long time.

11. Pay attention to your past injuries. If any part of your body is even close to hurting, drastically lower the weight and consider stopping the exercise or workout altogether.

12. Do not feel obligated to follow the journal exactly. If a movement is difficult for you for any reason (e.g. poor mobility, past injury, etc.), feel free to substitute that movement for one you are more comfortable with.

Holding Yourself Accountable
Staying Consistent

One of the best ways to continue doing this habit is to build it alongside a friend who is also passionate about becoming the best version of themself. Having someone to talk to and brainstorm about your specific pain points makes a huge difference. Their support (and sometimes competitive kick) can serve as a nice backup too.

Whether or not that person is also using this journal alongside you, you're still able to work together on establishing a consistent habit together.

If you're the type of person who benefits from a sense of community, we created a free Facebook group specifically designed to hold yourself accountable to using this journal, getting daily support, and for building habits in general.

There's daily activity on there and our team is extremely involved each day.

Join the Habit Nest accountability group here:
facebook.com/groups/habitnest

Commit.

No matter what happens tomorrow…

whether I am exhausted
*or have the **worst** day of my life…*

…whether I win the lottery
*or have the **best** day of my life…*

*I **<u>will</u>** do my workout.*

*My word is like **gold**.*

I will do whatever it takes
to make this happen.

I will workout at least this many times this week (circle one):

1   2   3   4   5   6   7

_____   _____
Signature   Date

The Workouts

Workout 1: Back & Triceps

DATE _____

1. ASSISTED PULL-UP

(ALTERNATIVE: PULL-UP OR TOWEL PULL)

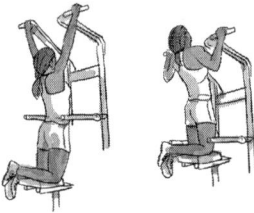

(Welcome to Workout 1! At first glance, many people may get overwhelmed here, but these workouts were designed to all be completed in 45mins – 1 hour.

That is the pace you should work to reach, with quick rests in between sets and focused, intense lifting with each exercise.)

SET 1	REPS: _____	(GOAL: TO FAILURE)	WEIGHT: _____
SET 2	REPS: _____	(GOAL: TO FAILURE)	WEIGHT: _____
SET 3	REPS: _____	(GOAL: TO FAILURE)	WEIGHT: _____
SET 4 (OPTIONAL)	REPS: _____	(GOAL: TO FAILURE)	WEIGHT: _____

2. T-BAR ROW

(ALTERNATIVE: UPPER BACK ROPE PULL)

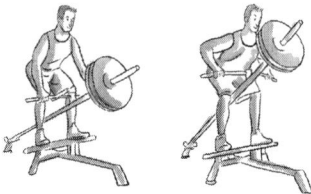

(Make sure to squeeze the muscles being worked at the climax of the movement and hold for 0.5–1 seconds; also, keep your chest on the pad to avoid compensating with other muscles.)

SET 1	REPS: _____	(GOAL: 10-15)	WEIGHT: _____
SET 2	REPS: _____	(GOAL: 8-12)	WEIGHT: _____
SET 3	REPS: _____	(GOAL: 6-8)	WEIGHT: _____
SET 4 (OPTIONAL)	REPS: _____	(GOAL: 4-6)	WEIGHT: _____

3. LAT PULLDOWN

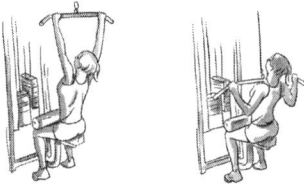

SET 1	REPS: _____	(GOAL: 10-15)	WEIGHT: _____
SET 2	REPS: _____	(GOAL: 8-12)	WEIGHT: _____
SET 3	REPS: _____	(GOAL: 6-8)	WEIGHT: _____
SET 4 (OPTIONAL)	REPS: _____	(GOAL: 4-6)	WEIGHT: _____

4. CLOSE GRIP CABLE ROW

(ALTERNATIVE: BENT OVER DUMBBELL ROW)

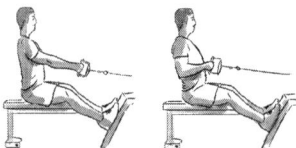

(Keep your back straight, not bent forward or backward, to make sure the lats bear the burden of the exercise. Keep your traps fully lowered!)

SET 1	REPS: _____	(GOAL: 10-15)	WEIGHT: _____
SET 2	REPS: _____	(GOAL: 8-12)	WEIGHT: _____
SET 3	REPS: _____	(GOAL: 6-8)	WEIGHT: _____
SET 4 (OPTIONAL)	REPS: _____	(GOAL: 4-6)	WEIGHT: _____

AMOUNT OF CARDIO DONE TODAY: _____

(Doing cardio is completely optional. If you do it, use the field to the left to track it using minutes, distance, or whatever metric you prefer.)

<u>Workout 1</u>: Back & **Triceps**

1. SKULL CRUSHER

(ALTERNATIVE: CLOSE GRIP BENCH PRESS OR
DUMBBELL PULLOVER)

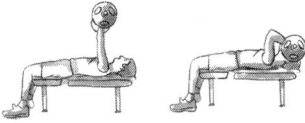

(Note: Anything not match up to your expectations for
your journal? Email us at support@habitnest.com so we
can make it right!)

SET 1	REPS: _____	(GOAL: 10-15)	WEIGHT: _____
SET 2	REPS: _____	(GOAL: 8-12)	WEIGHT: _____
SET 3	REPS: _____	(GOAL: 6-8)	WEIGHT: _____
SET 4 (OPTIONAL)	REPS: _____	(GOAL: 4-6)	WEIGHT: _____

2. OVERHEAD DUMBBELL EXTENSION

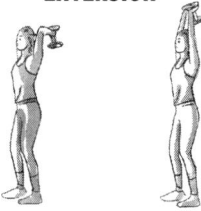

(Note: Mixing a pull-muscle (back) with a push-muscle (triceps) is
intended and will help engage multiple parts of your body together.)

SET 1	REPS: _____	(GOAL: 10-15)	WEIGHT: _____
SET 2	REPS: _____	(GOAL: 8-12)	WEIGHT: _____
SET 3	REPS: _____	(GOAL: 6-8)	WEIGHT: _____
SET 4 (OPTIONAL)	REPS: _____	(GOAL: 4-6)	WEIGHT: _____

3. ROPE PULLDOWN

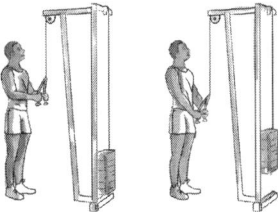

(Squeeze and hold for 0.5-1 seconds at the climax of the
movement -- when your arms straighten out.)

SET 1	REPS: _____	(GOAL: 10-15)	WEIGHT: _____
SET 2	REPS: _____	(GOAL: 8-12)	WEIGHT: _____
SET 3	REPS: _____	(GOAL: 6-8)	WEIGHT: _____
SET 4 (OPTIONAL)	REPS: _____	(GOAL: 4-6)	WEIGHT: _____

4. DIP

(ALTERNATIVE: ASSISTED DIP
OR SEATED DIP W/ MACHINE)

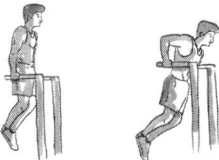

(Greyed sections are optional or won't apply to everybody!
For example, here you'd fill it in if you were adding
weights with a belt or using a seated/assisted dip machine.)

SET 1	REPS: _____	(GOAL: TO FAILURE)	WEIGHT: _____
SET 2	REPS: _____	(GOAL: TO FAILURE)	WEIGHT: _____
SET 3	REPS: _____	(GOAL: TO FAILURE)	WEIGHT: _____
SET 4 (OPTIONAL)	REPS: _____	(GOAL: TO FAILURE)	WEIGHT: _____

TODAY'S WORKOUT INTENSITY:
_____ / 10

Workout 2: Chest & Biceps

DATE _____

1. FLAT BENCH PRESS
(ALTERNATIVE: FLAT BENCH DUMBBELL PRESS)

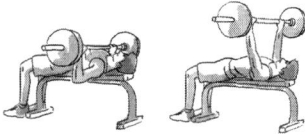

(Please use a spotter if you're unsure of whether you can complete one of your sets! Make sure to move faster on the way up, hold for 0.5 seconds, then slower on the way down.)

SET 1   REPS: _____ (GOAL: 10-15)   WEIGHT: _____

SET 2   REPS: _____ (GOAL: 8-12)   WEIGHT: _____

SET 3   REPS: _____ (GOAL: 6-8)   WEIGHT: _____

SET 4   REPS: _____ (GOAL: 4-6)   WEIGHT: _____
(OPTIONAL)

2. DECLINE BENCH PRESS

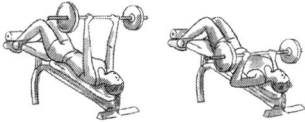

(Your goal rest times should be 30-120 seconds between each set/exercise, including the time it takes you to walk from one machine to another.)

SET 1   REPS: _____ (GOAL: 10-15)   WEIGHT: _____

SET 2   REPS: _____ (GOAL: 8-12)   WEIGHT: _____

SET 3   REPS: _____ (GOAL: 6-8)   WEIGHT: _____

SET 4   REPS: _____ (GOAL: 4-6)   WEIGHT: _____
(OPTIONAL)

3. INCLINE DUMBBELL PRESS
(ALTERNATIVE: INCLINE BENCH PRESS)

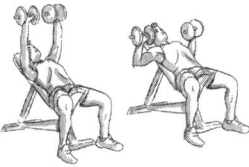

(To maximize the chest contraction and avoid using your shoulders too much, try to press the weights further out in front of you rather than on top of you.)

SET 1   REPS: _____ (GOAL: 10-15)   WEIGHT: _____

SET 2   REPS: _____ (GOAL: 8-12)   WEIGHT: _____

SET 3   REPS: _____ (GOAL: 6-8)   WEIGHT: _____

SET 4   REPS: _____ (GOAL: 4-6)   WEIGHT: _____
(OPTIONAL)

4. FLAT BENCH DUMBBELL FLY
(ALTERNATIVE: CHEST FLY W/ MACHINE)

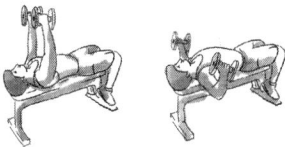

(Be very careful the first few times you do this - slowly bring the weights down to your sides. Make sure to move faster on the way up, squeeze your chest for 0.5-1 seconds, then move slower on the way down.)

SET 1   REPS: _____ (GOAL: 10-15)   WEIGHT: _____

SET 2   REPS: _____ (GOAL: 8-12)   WEIGHT: _____

SET 3   REPS: _____ (GOAL: 6-8)   WEIGHT: _____

SET 4   REPS: _____ (GOAL: 4-6)   WEIGHT: _____
(OPTIONAL)

AMOUNT OF CARDIO DONE TODAY:
_____

Workout 2: Chest & Biceps

1. PREACHER CURL

(ALTERNATIVE: SEATED DUMBBELL CURL)

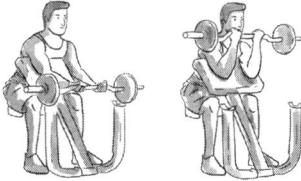

(You can also do this standing; the bench makes it harder to compensate by swinging your back. Try to move faster on the way up and slower on the way down to feel the resistance.)

SET 1   REPS: _____   (GOAL: 10-15)   WEIGHT: _____

SET 2   REPS: _____   (GOAL: 8-12)   WEIGHT: _____

SET 3   REPS: _____   (GOAL: 6-8)   WEIGHT: _____

SET 4   REPS: _____   (GOAL: 4-6)   WEIGHT: _____
[OPTIONAL]

2. DUMBBELL HAMMER CURL

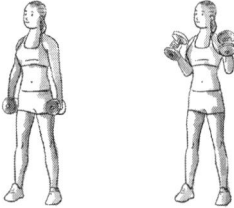

(Make sure your elbows are locked in place by your sides. The only movement should be your forearm going up and down. Try to move faster on the way up and slower on the way down.)

SET 1   REPS: _____   (GOAL: 10-15)   WEIGHT: _____

SET 2   REPS: _____   (GOAL: 8-12)   WEIGHT: _____

SET 3   REPS: _____   (GOAL: 6-8)   WEIGHT: _____

SET 4   REPS: _____   (GOAL: 4-6)   WEIGHT: _____
[OPTIONAL]

3. CONCENTRATION CURL

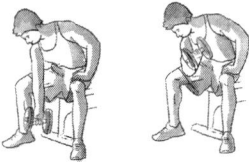

(Before you start, let your back find a comfortable position. Your elbow should stay still against your leg!)

SET 1   REPS: _____   (GOAL: 10-15)   WEIGHT: _____

SET 2   REPS: _____   (GOAL: 8-12)   WEIGHT: _____

SET 3   REPS: _____   (GOAL: 6-8)   WEIGHT: _____

SET 4   REPS: _____   (GOAL: 4-6)   WEIGHT: _____
[OPTIONAL]

4. OVERHEAD CABLE CURL

(ALTERNATIVE: DO ONE ARM AT A TIME)

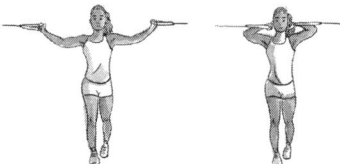

(Life hack: If you use this journal's elastic band to hold it closed, the band doubles up as a pen holder. Slide your pen clip through it, allowing your pen to rest on top of the book!)

SET 1   REPS: _____   (GOAL: 10-15)   WEIGHT: _____

SET 2   REPS: _____   (GOAL: 8-12)   WEIGHT: _____

SET 3   REPS: _____   (GOAL: 6-8)   WEIGHT: _____

SET 4   REPS: _____   (GOAL: 4-6)   WEIGHT: _____
[OPTIONAL]

TODAY'S WORKOUT INTENSITY:
_____ / 10

(Do your best to make each workout at least an 8 in intensity!)

Workout 3: Legs & Abs

DATE _____

1. LEG PRESS

(On leg days, if you're comfortable, include deadlifts and/ or squats with a barbell in place of any two exercises except for calves.)

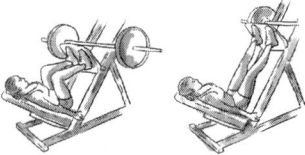

SET 1   REPS: _____   (GOAL: 10-15)   WEIGHT: _____

SET 2   REPS: _____   (GOAL: 8-12)   WEIGHT: _____

SET 3   REPS: _____   (GOAL: 6-8)   WEIGHT: _____

SET 4   REPS: _____   (GOAL: 4-6)   WEIGHT: _____
[OPTIONAL]

2. HACK SQUAT
(ALTERNATIVE: WEIGHTED LUNGE)

(The exercise index at the end of the journal includes detailed workout descriptions for all listed exercises, including 'alternative' ones.)

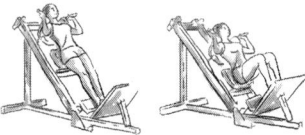

SET 1   REPS: _____   (GOAL: 10-15)   WEIGHT: _____

SET 2   REPS: _____   (GOAL: 8-12)   WEIGHT: _____

SET 3   REPS: _____   (GOAL: 6-8)   WEIGHT: _____

SET 4   REPS: _____   (GOAL: 4-6)   WEIGHT: _____
[OPTIONAL]

3. QUAD EXTENSION

(The goal is to progressively increase the weight on each set. Challenge yourself on EVERY set!)

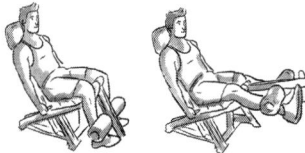

SET 1   REPS: _____   (GOAL: 10-15)   WEIGHT: _____

SET 2   REPS: _____   (GOAL: 8-12)   WEIGHT: _____

SET 3   REPS: _____   (GOAL: 6-8)   WEIGHT: _____

SET 4   REPS: _____   (GOAL: 4-6)   WEIGHT: _____
[OPTIONAL]

(If you really prefer not to do a given exercise, cross it out and put another in its place!)

4. HAMSTRING EXTENSION

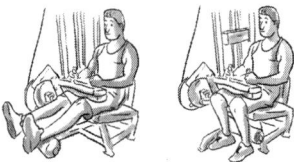

SET 1   REPS: _____   (GOAL: 10-15)   WEIGHT: _____

SET 2   REPS: _____   (GOAL: 8-12)   WEIGHT: _____

SET 3   REPS: _____   (GOAL: 6-8)   WEIGHT: _____

SET 4   REPS: _____   (GOAL: 4-6)   WEIGHT: _____
[OPTIONAL]

AMOUNT OF CARDIO DONE TODAY: _____

Workout 3: Legs & Abs

5. CALF RAISE
(ALTERNATIVE: SEATED CALF PRESS MACHINE)

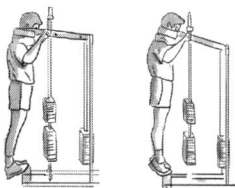

(Variation idea: Do 1/3rd of each set with your toes pointed straight, 1/3rd with your toes pointed away from each other, and 1/3rd with your toes pointed towards each other.)

SET 1   REPS: _____   (GOAL: 10-15)   WEIGHT: _____

SET 2   REPS: _____   (GOAL: 8-12)   WEIGHT: _____

SET 3   REPS: _____   (GOAL: 6-8)   WEIGHT: _____

SET 4   REPS: _____   (GOAL: 4-6)   WEIGHT: _____
(OPTIONAL)

1. KNEELING CABLE CRUNCH

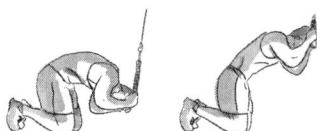

(Variation idea: Do 1/3rd of each set going straight down, 1/3rd going to your right side, and 1/3rd going to your left.)

SET 1   REPS: _____   (GOAL: 10-20)   WEIGHT: _____

SET 2   REPS: _____   (GOAL: 10-20)   WEIGHT: _____

SET 3   REPS: _____   (GOAL: 10-20)   WEIGHT: _____

2. LEG LIFT
(ALTERNATIVE: HANGING LEG LIFT)

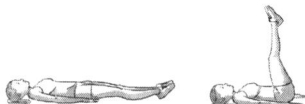

(You'll notice ab exercises only have three sets listed instead of four. This is because the abs are a smaller muscle and are mainly 'made in the kitchen' with good diet, requiring less of an exercise focus on them.)

SET 1   REPS: _____   (GOAL: 10-20)

SET 2   REPS: _____   (GOAL: 10-20)

SET 3   REPS: _____   (GOAL: 10-20)

3. STARFISH CRUNCH

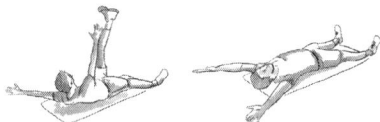

SET 1   REPS: _____   (GOAL: 10-20 EACH SIDE)

SET 2   REPS: _____   (GOAL: 10-20 EACH SIDE)

SET 3   REPS: _____   (GOAL: 10-20 EACH SIDE)

4. PLANK

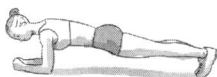

(Make sure to keep your back straight and your abdominal muscles and core locked tight.)

SET 1   TIME: _____   (GOAL: 45-90 SECONDS)

SET 2   TIME: _____   (GOAL: 45-90 SECONDS)

SET 3   TIME: _____   (GOAL: 45-90 SECONDS)

TODAY'S WORKOUT INTENSITY:
_____ / 10

Workout 4: Shoulders & Forearms

1. LATERAL DUMBBELL RAISE

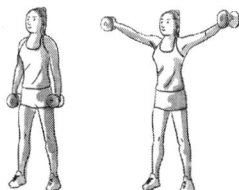

(Try your best to avoid swinging to get your arms up. This should be a controlled movement with your arms as straight as possible. Make sure to move faster on the way up, hold for 0.5 second, then slower on the way down.)

SET 1	REPS: _____	(GOAL: 10-15)	WEIGHT: _____
SET 2	REPS: _____	(GOAL: 8-12)	WEIGHT: _____
SET 3	REPS: _____	(GOAL: 6-8)	WEIGHT: _____
SET 4 (OPTIONAL)	REPS: _____	(GOAL: 4-6)	WEIGHT: _____

2. FRONT DUMBBELL RAISE

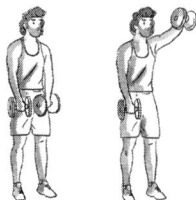

(Try the above tip for this exercise too!)

SET 1	REPS: _____	(GOAL: 10-15)	WEIGHT: _____
SET 2	REPS: _____	(GOAL: 8-12)	WEIGHT: _____
SET 3	REPS: _____	(GOAL: 6-8)	WEIGHT: _____
SET 4 (OPTIONAL)	REPS: _____	(GOAL: 4-6)	WEIGHT: _____

3. REVERSE FLY
(ALTERNATIVE: BENT OVER REAR DELT RAISE)

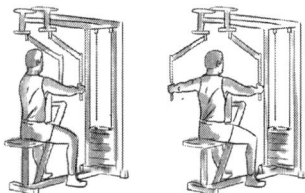

(The benefit of using machines is that they allow for the movement to be controlled while preventing you from compensating with other muscles.)

SET 1	REPS: _____	(GOAL: 10-15)	WEIGHT: _____
SET 2	REPS: _____	(GOAL: 8-12)	WEIGHT: _____
SET 3	REPS: _____	(GOAL: 6-8)	WEIGHT: _____
SET 4 (OPTIONAL)	REPS: _____	(GOAL: 4-6)	WEIGHT: _____

4. SEATED DUMBBELL PRESS

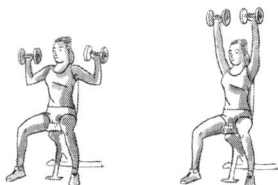

(Your arms should be at a 90-degree angle with the weights parallel to the ground; you don't want your arms to cave in or fall outward. Make sure to move faster on the way up, slower on the way down, and then hold before you repeat!)

SET 1	REPS: _____	(GOAL: 10-15)	WEIGHT: _____
SET 2	REPS: _____	(GOAL: 8-12)	WEIGHT: _____
SET 3	REPS: _____	(GOAL: 6-8)	WEIGHT: _____
SET 4 (OPTIONAL)	REPS: _____	(GOAL: 4-6)	WEIGHT: _____

AMOUNT OF CARDIO DONE TODAY:
_____

56

Workout 4: Shoulders & Forearms

5. SHRUG

(Make sure you stand straight up, hold the weights comfortably in your hands, and simply pull your shoulders up and down. This muscle grows fairly quickly.)

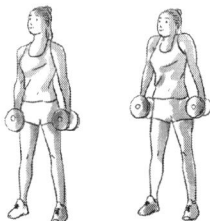

SET 1	REPS: _____	(GOAL: 10-15)	WEIGHT: _____
SET 2	REPS: _____	(GOAL: 8-12)	WEIGHT: _____
SET 3	REPS: _____	(GOAL: 6-8)	WEIGHT: _____
SET 4 [OPTIONAL]	REPS: _____	(GOAL: 4-6)	WEIGHT: _____

1. REVERSE GRIP EZ BAR CURL
(ALTERNATIVE: REVERSE GRIP CURL W/ DUMBBELLS)

(Make sure to keep your elbows in place. This exercise primarily works the front part of your forearm; you can also do this standing.)

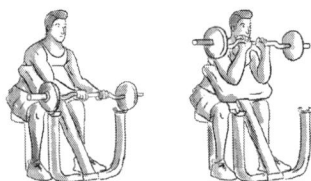

SET 1	REPS: _____	(GOAL: 10-15)	WEIGHT: _____
SET 2	REPS: _____	(GOAL: 8-12)	WEIGHT: _____
SET 3	REPS: _____	(GOAL: 6-8)	WEIGHT: _____
SET 4 [OPTIONAL]	REPS: _____	(GOAL: 4-6)	WEIGHT: _____

2. BARBELL TWIST-UP
(ALTERNATIVE: BARBELL TWIST-UP W/ DUMBBELLS)

(In this exercise, simply roll your wrists up and down. This primarily works the back part of your forearm.)

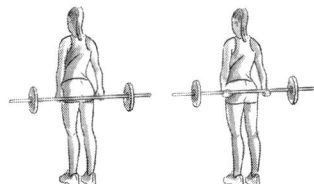

SET 1	REPS: _____	(GOAL: 10-15)	WEIGHT: _____
SET 2	REPS: _____	(GOAL: 8-12)	WEIGHT: _____
SET 3	REPS: _____	(GOAL: 6-8)	WEIGHT: _____
SET 4 [OPTIONAL]	REPS: _____	(GOAL: 4-6)	WEIGHT: _____

TODAY'S WORKOUT INTENSITY:
_____ / 10

Workout 5: Full Body Circuit

DATE _____

*Rest for **15-20 seconds** between each exercise, then rest for **1-2 minutes** after completing the entire circuit. Complete the full circuit **a total of 4-5 times.***

1. JUMPING JACKS

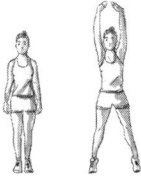

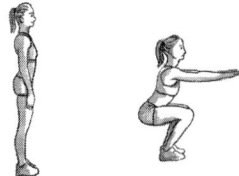

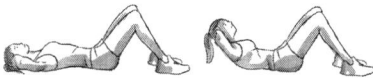

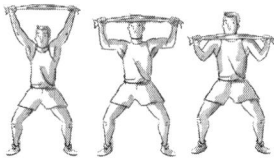

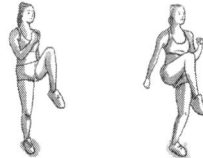

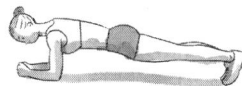

(Duration: 30 Seconds)

2. AIR SQUAT

(Duration: 30 Seconds)

3. CRUNCH

(Duration: 30 Seconds)

4. MOUNTAIN CLIMBER

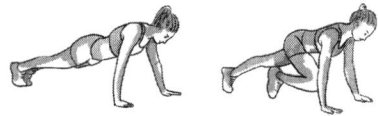

(Duration: 30 Seconds)

5. TOWEL PULL

(Duration: 30 Seconds)

6. HIGH KNEE

(Duration: 30 Seconds)

7. IN AND OUT PUSH-UP

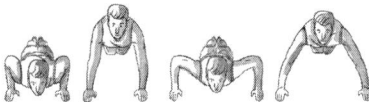

(Duration: 30 Seconds)

8. PLANK

(Duration: 30 Seconds)

TODAY'S WORKOUT INTENSITY:
_____ / 10

Double Pro-Tip

Create a phone ritual when going to the gym.

When your phone is on and in your pocket as you workout, it's a ticking time-bomb of distraction. As Arnold Schwarzenegger stated,

"When I see people texting in the gym, they're not serious. This is Mickey Mouse stuff. You train, or you don't."

You need to conquer your phone and its infinite distracting glory at the gym. This works best by creating a ritual with your phone when you arrive.

Aside from being mindful of not using it, you can decrease the amount of distractions it provides by performing the following:

1. *Set your phone in airplane mode, or airplane mode and wi-fi on if you're using it to stream music / audiobooks.*
2. *Turn on "do not disturb" mode.*
3. *Set your phone to grayscale mode (makes a huge difference). Google how to do this and set it up as a shortcut on your phone.*

Pack for the gym the night before.

By starting your day with everything you need to get going, you'll feel prepared, organized, and ready to take on your day with momentum!

Packing your gym clothes and bag will help hold you accountable for actually going to the gym that day as well.

This tip is even more effective if you work out early in the mornings as you're able to get up and move!

Pssssstt... We like rewarding people (like you) who TAKE ACTION and actually use this journal.

Email us now at secret+lifting@habitnest.com for a secret gift ;)

Workout 6: Back & Shoulders

1. LAT PULLDOWN

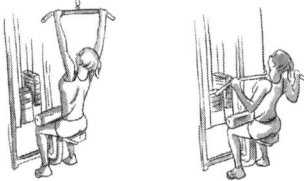

(Before starting your workout each day, go back and fill in the 'Previous Best' sections for all exercises that day.)

PREVIOUS BEST
(WORKOUT 1)

REPS: _____   WEIGHT: _____

SET 1 REPS: _____ (GOAL: 10-15) WEIGHT: _____

SET 2 REPS: _____ (GOAL: 8-12) WEIGHT: _____

SET 3 REPS: _____ (GOAL: 6-8) WEIGHT: _____

SET 4 REPS: _____ (GOAL: 4-6) WEIGHT: _____
(OPTIONAL)

2. BENT OVER DUMBBELL ROW
(ALTERNATIVE: CLOSE GRIP CABLE ROW)

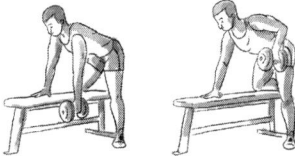

(Make sure to keep your back straight. When doing the movement, try to keep your elbow as close to your body as possible to feel your lat and upper back contract.)

SET 1 REPS: _____ (GOAL: 10-15) WEIGHT: _____

SET 2 REPS: _____ (GOAL: 8-12) WEIGHT: _____

SET 3 REPS: _____ (GOAL: 6-8) WEIGHT: _____

SET 4 REPS: _____ (GOAL: 4-6) WEIGHT: _____
(OPTIONAL)

3. STRAIGHT ARM PULLDOWN

(Your arms should stay straight to avoid doing a tricep pulldown. Try to push your butt and hips back and out, keep your back straight, and pull the rope with your arms straight down.)

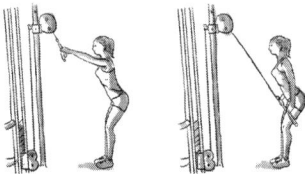

SET 1 REPS: _____ (GOAL: 10-15) WEIGHT: _____

SET 2 REPS: _____ (GOAL: 8-12) WEIGHT: _____

SET 3 REPS: _____ (GOAL: 6-8) WEIGHT: _____

SET 4 REPS: _____ (GOAL: 4-6) WEIGHT: _____
(OPTIONAL)

4. T-BAR ROW
(ALTERNATIVE: UPPER BACK ROPE PULL)

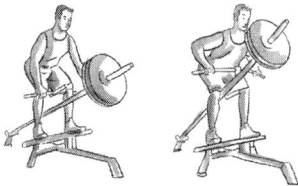

(If you do an 'Alternative' exercise instead of the designated one, circle it so you know what you completed when flipping back for reference.)

PREVIOUS BEST
(WORKOUT 1)

REPS: _____   WEIGHT: _____

SET 1 REPS: _____ (GOAL: 10-15) WEIGHT: _____

SET 2 REPS: _____ (GOAL: 8-12) WEIGHT: _____

SET 3 REPS: _____ (GOAL: 6-8) WEIGHT: _____

SET 4 REPS: _____ (GOAL: 4-6) WEIGHT: _____
(OPTIONAL)

AMOUNT OF CARDIO DONE TODAY:
_____

<u>Workout 6:</u> Back & <u>Shoulders</u>

1. LATERAL DUMBBELL RAISE

PREVIOUS BEST
(WORKOUT 4)

(You can also do this with one arm at a time.)

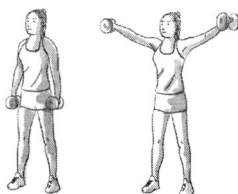

REPS: _____ WEIGHT: _____

SET 1 REPS: _____ (GOAL: 10-15) WEIGHT: _____

SET 2 REPS: _____ (GOAL: 8-12) WEIGHT: _____

SET 3 REPS: _____ (GOAL: 6-8) WEIGHT: _____

SET 4 REPS: _____ (GOAL: 4-6) WEIGHT: _____
(OPTIONAL)

2. FRONT DUMBBELL RAISE

(You can also do this with one arm at a time.)

PREVIOUS BEST
(WORKOUT 4)

REPS: _____ WEIGHT: _____

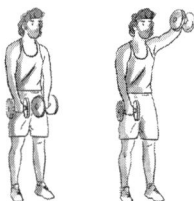

SET 1 REPS: _____ (GOAL: 10-15) WEIGHT: _____

SET 2 REPS: _____ (GOAL: 8-12) WEIGHT: _____

SET 3 REPS: _____ (GOAL: 6-8) WEIGHT: _____

SET 4 REPS: _____ (GOAL: 4-6) WEIGHT: _____
(OPTIONAL)

(Although we included set rep ranges to follow for each exercise, if you still have 'more in you' when you reach the upper range of an exercise, feel free to keep going and reach failure.)

3. REVERSE FLY

(ALTERNATIVE: BENT OVER REAR DELT RAISE)

PREVIOUS BEST
(WORKOUT 4)

REPS: _____ WEIGHT: _____

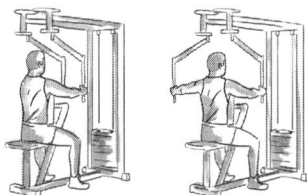

SET 1 REPS: _____ (GOAL: 10-15) WEIGHT: _____

SET 2 REPS: _____ (GOAL: 8-12) WEIGHT: _____

SET 3 REPS: _____ (GOAL: 6-8) WEIGHT: _____

SET 4 REPS: _____ (GOAL: 4-6) WEIGHT: _____
(OPTIONAL)

4. ARNOLD DUMBBELL PRESS

(ALTERNATIVE: SEATED DUMBBELL PRESS)

(This is just like doing the dumbbell press, only at the bottom, you twist your hands so they're facing you and twist them back as you lift up. It might be smart to use a lighter weight when you're first starting since this exercise can be a little bit more difficult.)

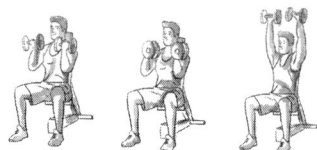

SET 1 REPS: _____ (GOAL: 10-15) WEIGHT: _____

SET 2 REPS: _____ (GOAL: 8-12) WEIGHT: _____

SET 3 REPS: _____ (GOAL: 6-8) WEIGHT: _____

SET 4 REPS: _____ (GOAL: 4-6) WEIGHT: _____
(OPTIONAL)

TODAY'S WORKOUT INTENSITY:
_____ / 10

Common Form Issue: **Biceps**

Problem

You're swinging your back backwards towards the second half of the movement.

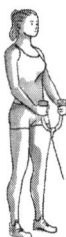

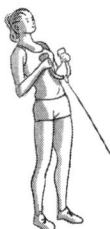

Improper Form

How to Fix This

Keep your back stationary and upright - do not move it. If you can't complete the movement like that, go down in weight to strengthen your muscles first.

Note: You may feel some of the muscles in your upper back (specifically the erector spinae) being worked if they're underdeveloped as a supporting muscle.

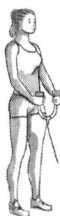

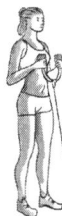

Proper Form

Exercises This Concept Applies To

All Bicep Exercises!

Common Form Issue: **Triceps**

(X) ***Problem***

Your wrists bend during movements to help move the weight.

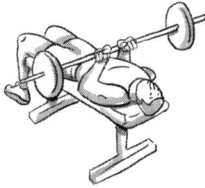

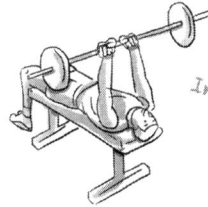

Improper Form

(✓) ***How to Fix This***

Imagine a metal rod is going through your arm, your wrist, and up to your fingers. Don't allow any bending to occur throughout the movement.

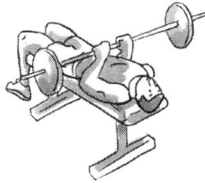

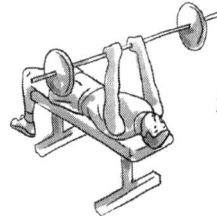

Proper Form

Exercises This Concept Applies To

Skull Crusher, Close Grip Bench Press

Workout 7: Biceps & Triceps

DATE _____

1. PREACHER CURL
(ALTERNATIVE: SEATED DUMBBELL CURL)

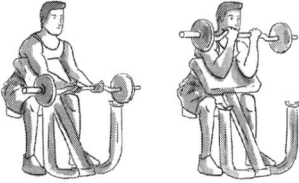

PREVIOUS BEST (WORKOUT 2)

(Fill in your reps/weight used on your last set (Set 3 or 4) for all 'Previous Best' sections.)

REPS: _____   WEIGHT: _____

SET 1 REPS: _____ (GOAL: 10-15) WEIGHT: _____
SET 2 REPS: _____ (GOAL: 8-12) WEIGHT: _____
SET 3 REPS: _____ (GOAL: 6-8) WEIGHT: _____
SET 4 REPS: _____ (GOAL: 4-6) WEIGHT: _____
(OPTIONAL)

2. ROPE HAMMER CURL

(Make sure your elbows stay still, just like you're doing hammer curls.)

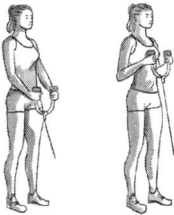

SET 1 REPS: _____ (GOAL: 10-15) WEIGHT: _____
SET 2 REPS: _____ (GOAL: 8-12) WEIGHT: _____
SET 3 REPS: _____ (GOAL: 6-8) WEIGHT: _____
SET 4 REPS: _____ (GOAL: 4-6) WEIGHT: _____
(OPTIONAL)

3. ZOTTMAN CURL

(Feel the burn! This exercise is an ordinary curl on the way up, then you twist your weights and do a hammer curl on the way down.)

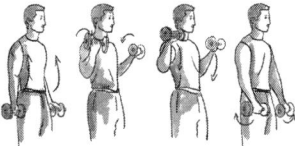

SET 1 REPS: _____ (GOAL: 10-15) WEIGHT: _____
SET 2 REPS: _____ (GOAL: 8-12) WEIGHT: _____
SET 3 REPS: _____ (GOAL: 6-8) WEIGHT: _____
SET 4 REPS: _____ (GOAL: 4-6) WEIGHT: _____
(OPTIONAL)

4. UNDERHAND CABLE CURL

(You can also do this standing with individual cables in each hand.)

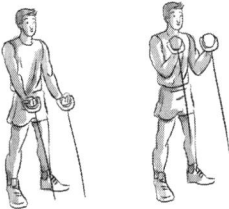

SET 1 REPS: _____ (GOAL: 10-15) WEIGHT: _____
SET 2 REPS: _____ (GOAL: 8-12) WEIGHT: _____
SET 3 REPS: _____ (GOAL: 6-8) WEIGHT: _____
SET 4 REPS: _____ (GOAL: 4-6) WEIGHT: _____
(OPTIONAL)

AMOUNT OF CARDIO DONE TODAY: _____

<u>Workout 7</u>: Biceps & **Triceps**

1. SKULL CRUSHER

(ALTERNATIVE: STRAIGHT BAR PULLDOWN)

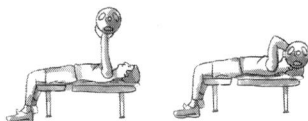

(Make sure to keep your elbows locked in and your wrists straight like a rod through your forearm and out your hand!)

PREVIOUS BEST
(WORKOUT 1)   REPS: _____   WEIGHT: _____

SET 1   REPS: _____   (GOAL: 10-15)   WEIGHT: _____

SET 2   REPS: _____   (GOAL: 8-12)   WEIGHT: _____

SET 3   REPS: _____   (GOAL: 6-8)   WEIGHT: _____

SET 4   REPS: _____   (GOAL: 4-6)   WEIGHT: _____
(OPTIONAL)

2. CLOSE GRIP BENCH PRESS

(ALTERNATIVE: OVERHEAD DUMBBELL EXTENSION)

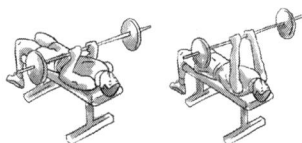

(Make sure to keep your hands close together and your wrists straight. Move faster on the way up and slower on the way down.)

SET 1   REPS: _____   (GOAL: 10-15)   WEIGHT: _____

SET 2   REPS: _____   (GOAL: 8-12)   WEIGHT: _____

SET 3   REPS: _____   (GOAL: 6-8)   WEIGHT: _____

SET 4   REPS: _____   (GOAL: 4-6)   WEIGHT: _____
(OPTIONAL)

(Feel free to add in descriptive notes for yourself to keep in mind, e.g. 'too easy' or 'too heavy' for the weights you chose. This can help you choose the proper starting / goal weights for future exercises.)

3. ROPE PULLDOWN

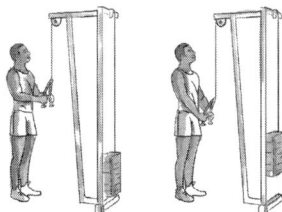

PREVIOUS BEST
(WORKOUT 1)   REPS: _____   WEIGHT: _____

SET 1   REPS: _____   (GOAL: 10-15)   WEIGHT: _____

SET 2   REPS: _____   (GOAL: 8-12)   WEIGHT: _____

SET 3   REPS: _____   (GOAL: 6-8)   WEIGHT: _____

SET 4   REPS: _____   (GOAL: 4-6)   WEIGHT: _____
(OPTIONAL)

4. DIP

(ALTERNATIVE: ASSISTED DIP OR SEATED DIP W/ MACHINE)

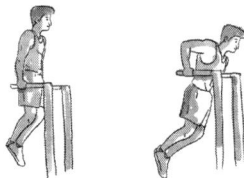

(If it's difficult at first, use the assisted dip machine! Make sure to move slower on the way down and faster on the way up.)

PREVIOUS BEST
(WORKOUT 1)   REPS: _____   WEIGHT: _____

SET 1   REPS: _____   (GOAL: TO FAILURE)   WEIGHT: _____

SET 2   REPS: _____   (GOAL: TO FAILURE)   WEIGHT: _____

SET 3   REPS: _____   (GOAL: TO FAILURE)   WEIGHT: _____

SET 4   REPS: _____   (GOAL: TO FAILURE)   WEIGHT: _____
(OPTIONAL)

TODAY'S WORKOUT INTENSITY:
_____ / 10

Workout 8: Chest & Forearms

DATE _____

1. FLAT BENCH PRESS

(ALTERNATIVE: FLAT BENCH DUMBBELL PRESS)

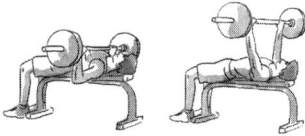

PREVIOUS BEST (WORKOUT 2)   REPS: _____   WEIGHT: _____

SET 1   REPS: _____ (GOAL: 10-15)   WEIGHT: _____

SET 2   REPS: _____ (GOAL: 8-12)   WEIGHT: _____

SET 3   REPS: _____ (GOAL: 6-8)   WEIGHT: _____

SET 4 (OPTIONAL)   REPS: _____ (GOAL: 4-6)   WEIGHT: _____

(It might take some time getting used to this position. The bar should be parallel to the bottom of your chest as it comes down.)

2. DECLINE BENCH PRESS

(ALTERNATIVE: HIGH TO LOW CABLE FLY)

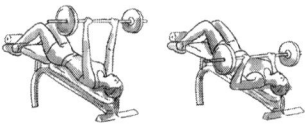

PREVIOUS BEST (WORKOUT 2)   REPS: _____   WEIGHT: _____

SET 1   REPS: _____ (GOAL: 10-15)   WEIGHT: _____

SET 2   REPS: _____ (GOAL: 8-12)   WEIGHT: _____

SET 3   REPS: _____ (GOAL: 6-8)   WEIGHT: _____

SET 4 (OPTIONAL)   REPS: _____ (GOAL: 4-6)   WEIGHT: _____

(Even if you have past experience doing these exercises, that doesn't necessarily mean they've been done correctly. We cover the little nuances with each exercise that separates good from bad form in the index - we recommend reading the whole thing.)

3. INCLINE DUMBBELL PRESS

(ALTERNATIVE: INCLINE BENCH PRESS)

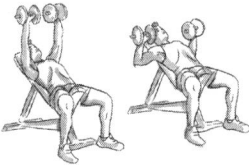

PREVIOUS BEST (WORKOUT 2)   REPS: _____   WEIGHT: _____

SET 1   REPS: _____ (GOAL: 10-15)   WEIGHT: _____

SET 2   REPS: _____ (GOAL: 8-12)   WEIGHT: _____

SET 3   REPS: _____ (GOAL: 6-8)   WEIGHT: _____

SET 4 (OPTIONAL)   REPS: _____ (GOAL: 4-6)   WEIGHT: _____

4. INCLINE DUMBBELL FLY

(Make sure to be very careful with this exercise as you open your arms slowly while keeping them slightly bent. Try to squeeze your chest when your arms come together at the top.)

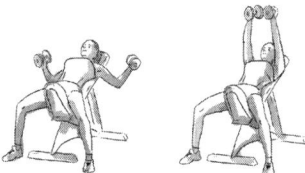

SET 1   REPS: _____ (GOAL: 10-15)   WEIGHT: _____

SET 2   REPS: _____ (GOAL: 8-12)   WEIGHT: _____

SET 3   REPS: _____ (GOAL: 6-8)   WEIGHT: _____

SET 4 (OPTIONAL)   REPS: _____ (GOAL: 4-6)   WEIGHT: _____

AMOUNT OF CARDIO DONE TODAY:
_____

66

Workout 8: Chest & Forearms

5. CABLE CROSSOVER

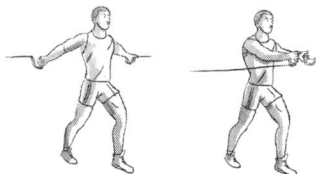

(Make sure to keep your arms straight with a slight bend in your elbows as you pull your hands together. Squeeze your chest when your hands come together and slowly open your arms to feel the resistance.)

SET 1	REPS: _____ (GOAL: 10-15)	WEIGHT: _____
SET 2	REPS: _____ (GOAL: 8-12)	WEIGHT: _____
SET 3	REPS: _____ (GOAL: 6-8)	WEIGHT: _____
SET 4 (OPTIONAL)	REPS: _____ (GOAL: 4-6)	WEIGHT: _____

1. REVERSE GRIP EZ BAR CURL
(ALTERNATIVE: FARMER'S WALK)

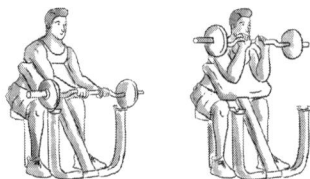

(If you are supersetting between two machines, you can use this physical journal to show that you are using a machine. That said, always be mindful of others and try to share / work in whenever possible.)

PREVIOUS BEST (WORKOUT 4)   REPS: _____   WEIGHT: _____

SET 1	REPS: _____ (GOAL: 10-15)	WEIGHT: _____
SET 2	REPS: _____ (GOAL: 8-12)	WEIGHT: _____
SET 3	REPS: _____ (GOAL: 6-8)	WEIGHT: _____
SET 4 (OPTIONAL)	REPS: _____ (GOAL: 4-6)	WEIGHT: _____

2. BARBELL TWIST-UP
(ALTERNATIVE: PULL-UP BAR HANG)

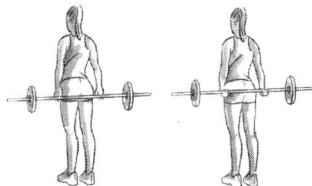

(You don't have to wait until you feel ready to begin each new set. Try starting sets even when it doesn't feel naturally right to push yourself and maintain a high level of intensity.)

PREVIOUS BEST (WORKOUT 4)   REPS: _____   WEIGHT: _____

SET 1	REPS: _____ (GOAL: 10-15)	WEIGHT: _____
SET 2	REPS: _____ (GOAL: 8-12)	WEIGHT: _____
SET 3	REPS: _____ (GOAL: 6-8)	WEIGHT: _____
SET 4 (OPTIONAL)	REPS: _____ (GOAL: 4-6)	WEIGHT: _____

TODAY'S WORKOUT INTENSITY:
_____ / 10

Workout 9: Legs & Abs

DATE _____

1. DEADLIFT
(ALTERNATIVE: LEG PRESS)

(When working with heavier compound movements like the deadlift and squat, exercise extra caution to avoid injury. Never push through pain and listen to your body.)

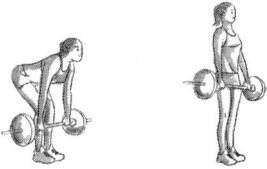

SET 1   REPS: _____ (GOAL: 10-15)   WEIGHT: _____

SET 2   REPS: _____ (GOAL: 8-12)   WEIGHT: _____

SET 3   REPS: _____ (GOAL: 6-8)   WEIGHT: _____

SET 4   REPS: _____ (GOAL: 4-6)   WEIGHT: _____
(OPTIONAL)

2. BARBELL SQUAT
(ALTERNATIVE: HACK SQUAT)

(Properly performing the squat requires great mobility. Spend time improving yours as it will not only help you avoid injury but also set you up to lift as heavily as possible.)

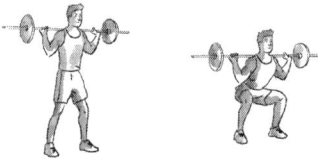

SET 1   REPS: _____ (GOAL: 10-15)   WEIGHT: _____

SET 2   REPS: _____ (GOAL: 8-12)   WEIGHT: _____

SET 3   REPS: _____ (GOAL: 6-8)   WEIGHT: _____

SET 4   REPS: _____ (GOAL: 4-6)   WEIGHT: _____
(OPTIONAL)

3. QUAD EXTENSION
(ALTERNATIVE: WEIGHTED LUNGE)

(Filling out the 'Previous Best' section is very important, as it sets a clear goal for you to beat and lets you see the progress you're making after each workout.)

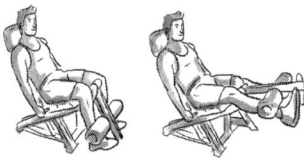

PREVIOUS BEST   REPS: _____   WEIGHT: _____
(WORKOUT 3)

SET 1   REPS: _____ (GOAL: 10-15)   WEIGHT: _____

SET 2   REPS: _____ (GOAL: 8-12)   WEIGHT: _____

SET 3   REPS: _____ (GOAL: 6-8)   WEIGHT: _____

SET 4   REPS: _____ (GOAL: 4-6)   WEIGHT: _____
(OPTIONAL)

4. HAMSTRING EXTENSION

(As you encounter new exercises in the journal, experiment with different, safe weight ranges to learn what works best for you over time.)

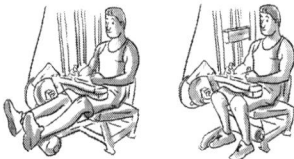

PREVIOUS BEST   REPS: _____   WEIGHT: _____
(WORKOUT 3)

SET 1   REPS: _____ (GOAL: 10-15)   WEIGHT: _____

SET 2   REPS: _____ (GOAL: 8-12)   WEIGHT: _____

SET 3   REPS: _____ (GOAL: 6-8)   WEIGHT: _____

SET 4   REPS: _____ (GOAL: 4-6)   WEIGHT: _____
(OPTIONAL)

AMOUNT OF CARDIO DONE TODAY: _____

Workout 9: Legs & Abs

5. CALF RAISE

(ALTERNATIVE: SEATED CALF PRESS MACHINE)

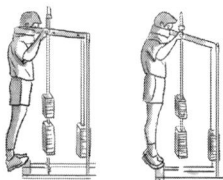

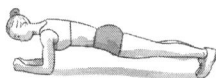

PREVIOUS BEST (WORKOUT 3)	REPS: _____		WEIGHT: _____
SET 1	REPS: _____	(GOAL: 10-15)	WEIGHT: _____
SET 2	REPS: _____	(GOAL: 8-12)	WEIGHT: _____
SET 3	REPS: _____	(GOAL: 6-8)	WEIGHT: _____
SET 4 (OPTIONAL)	REPS: _____	(GOAL: 4-6)	WEIGHT: _____

1. KNEELING CABLE CRUNCH

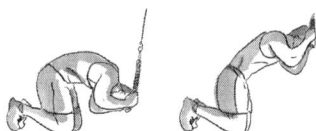

PREVIOUS BEST (WORKOUT 3)	REPS: _____		WEIGHT: _____
SET 1	REPS: _____	(GOAL: 10-20)	WEIGHT: _____
SET 2	REPS: _____	(GOAL: 10-20)	WEIGHT: _____
SET 3	REPS: _____	(GOAL: 10-20)	WEIGHT: _____

2. HANGING LEG LIFT

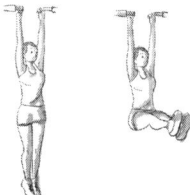

SET 1	REPS: _____	(GOAL: 10-20)
SET 2	REPS: _____	(GOAL: 10-20)
SET 3	REPS: _____	(GOAL: 10-20)

3. BICYCLE CRUNCH

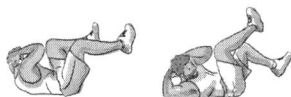

SET 1	REPS: _____	(GOAL: 10-20 EACH SIDE)
SET 2	REPS: _____	(GOAL: 10-20 EACH SIDE)
SET 3	REPS: _____	(GOAL: 10-20 EACH SIDE)

4. PLANK

PREVIOUS BEST (WORKOUT 3)	TIME: _____	
SET 1	TIME: _____	(GOAL: 45-90 SECONDS)
SET 2	TIME: _____	(GOAL: 45-90 SECONDS)
SET 3	TIME: _____	(GOAL: 45-90 SECONDS)

TODAY'S WORKOUT INTENSITY:
_____ / 10

Workout 10: Full Body Circuit

*Rest for **15-20 seconds** between each exercise, then rest for **1-2 minutes** after completing the entire circuit. Complete the full circuit **a total of 4-5 times.***

1. RUN IN PLACE

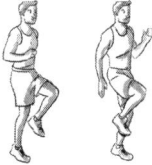

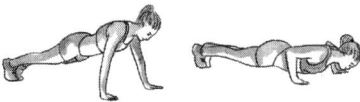

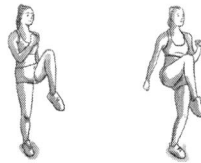

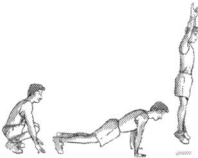

(Duration: 30 Seconds)

2. ALTERNATING LUNGE

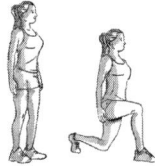

(Duration: 30 Seconds)

3. STARFISH CRUNCH

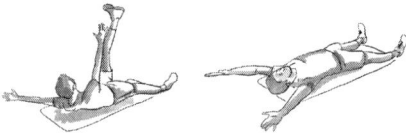

(Duration: 30 Seconds)

4. TOWEL SNATCH

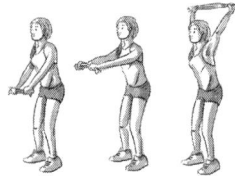

(Duration: 30 Seconds)

5. PUSH-UP

(Duration: 30 Seconds)

6. HIGH KNEE

(Duration: 30 Seconds)

7. BURPEE

(Duration: 30 Seconds)

8. BICYCLE CRUNCH

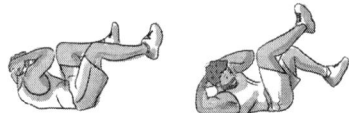

(Duration: 30 Seconds)

TODAY'S WORKOUT INTENSITY:
_____ / 10

<u>Check-In</u> ⊘

Taking a few minutes to simply STOP and evaluate how you're doing mentally, physically, and emotionally every few weeks of a training program can be extremely helpful to your experience with it.

Take a few minutes to answer the following questions with honesty!

What do I expect out of this process? How do I want to look? Feel?

_____

_____

_____

_____

How am I feeling about the quality and intensity of my workouts?

_____

_____

_____

_____

How do I feel about the way I look?

_____

_____

_____

_____

What do I want to learn more about (e.g. muscle anatomy, nutrition, mobility, etc.) that I can spend some time researching?

_____

_____

_____

_____

Bonus Challenge

> *Achieve a deep mind-muscle connection with every single rep you perform.*

We talked about the scientific importance of having mind-muscle connection in the intro of this journal, but it is so imperative (and so easy to misunderstand) that it's worth repeating here.

Many people understand mind-muscle connection as simply 'being focused' and 'not being distracted' during workouts. Although that's part of it, the true effectiveness of mind-muscle connection comes when you:

1. **Turn off all other muscles that are not part of the movement.** Only lift the weight using the specific muscles needed for it.

2. **Keep the muscle(s) you're using fully engaged, flexed, and isolated the entire time** throughout each movement. For every second of every rep.

To take this concept to the next level, you should isolate and flex the specific muscle you're going to use before every single exercise so you'll know exactly what to activate with each rep.

This means at the top or bottom of each rep, you keep your muscle engaged and fully lifting the weight as you would in the middle of a rep.

You may have to drastically drop in weight to do this, which is a sign you're doing a substantial amount of 'cheating reps' and leaving lots of a movement's primary muscles barely used.

You should also be prepared to know what muscles can help you break form and cheat so you can be extra vigilant of not using them.

Play around with this concept during your next workout if it's new for you and see if you notice a big difference.

<u>Workout 11: Back & Abs</u>

DATE _____

(Bonus: You can further strengthen your grip by hanging on the pull-up bar for as long as you can after completing your last rep.)

1. ASSISTED PULL-UP
(ALTERNATIVE: PULL-UP OR TOWEL PULL)

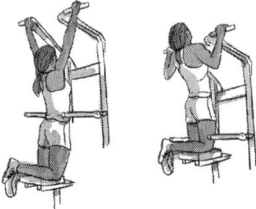

PREVIOUS BEST (WORKOUT 1)   REPS: _____   WEIGHT: _____

SET 1   REPS: _____ (GOAL: 10-15)   WEIGHT: _____
SET 2   REPS: _____ (GOAL: 8-12)   WEIGHT: _____
SET 3   REPS: _____ (GOAL: 6-8)   WEIGHT: _____
SET 4 (OPTIONAL)   REPS: _____ (GOAL: 4-6)   WEIGHT: _____

(Note: You'll never fully feel ready to move up in weight — challenge yourself safely and find out.)

2. CLOSE GRIP CABLE ROW
(ALTERNATIVE: BENT OVER DUMBBELL ROW)

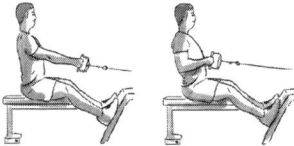

PREVIOUS BEST (WORKOUT 1)   REPS: _____   WEIGHT: _____

SET 1   REPS: _____ (GOAL: 10-15)   WEIGHT: _____
SET 2   REPS: _____ (GOAL: 8-12)   WEIGHT: _____
SET 3   REPS: _____ (GOAL: 6-8)   WEIGHT: _____
SET 4 (OPTIONAL)   REPS: _____ (GOAL: 4-6)   WEIGHT: _____

3. STRAIGHT ARM PULLDOWN

PREVIOUS BEST (WORKOUT 6)   REPS: _____   WEIGHT: _____

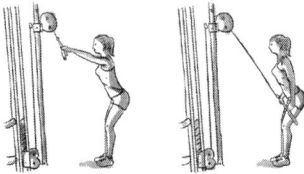

SET 1   REPS: _____ (GOAL: 10-15)   WEIGHT: _____
SET 2   REPS: _____ (GOAL: 8-12)   WEIGHT: _____
SET 3   REPS: _____ (GOAL: 6-8)   WEIGHT: _____
SET 4 (OPTIONAL)   REPS: _____ (GOAL: 4-6)   WEIGHT: _____

4. REVERSE GRIP LAT PULLDOWN

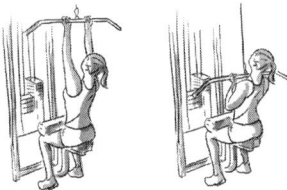

SET 1   REPS: _____ (GOAL: 10-15)   WEIGHT: _____
SET 2   REPS: _____ (GOAL: 8-12)   WEIGHT: _____
SET 3   REPS: _____ (GOAL: 6-8)   WEIGHT: _____
SET 4 (OPTIONAL)   REPS: _____ (GOAL: 4-6)   WEIGHT: _____

AMOUNT OF CARDIO DONE TODAY: _____

74

Workout 11: Back & Abs

5. T-BAR ROW

(ALTERNATIVE: BENT OVER DUMBBELL ROW)

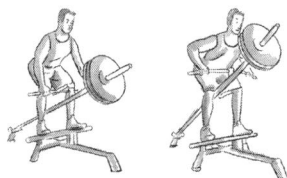

PREVIOUS BEST (WORKOUT 6)   REPS: _____   WEIGHT: _____

SET 1   REPS: _____   (GOAL: 10-15)   WEIGHT: _____

SET 2   REPS: _____   (GOAL: 8-12)   WEIGHT: _____

SET 3   REPS: _____   (GOAL: 6-8)   WEIGHT: _____

SET 4 (OPTIONAL)   REPS: _____   (GOAL: 4-6)   WEIGHT: _____

1. KNEELING CABLE CRUNCH

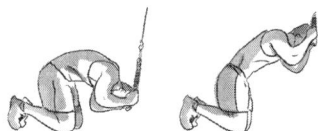

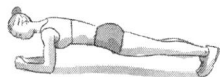

PREVIOUS BEST (WORKOUT 9)   REPS: _____   WEIGHT: _____

SET 1   REPS: _____   (GOAL: 10-20)   WEIGHT: _____

SET 2   REPS: _____   (GOAL: 10-20)   WEIGHT: _____

SET 3   REPS: _____   (GOAL: 10-20)   WEIGHT: _____

2. LEG LIFT

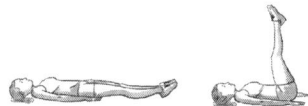

PREVIOUS BEST (WORKOUT 3)   REPS: _____

SET 1   REPS: _____   (GOAL: 10-20)

SET 2   REPS: _____   (GOAL: 10-20)

SET 3   REPS: _____   (GOAL: 10-20)

3. RUSSIAN TWIST

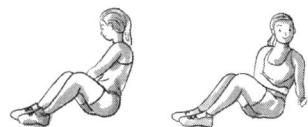

SET 1   REPS: _____   (GOAL: 10-20 EACH SIDE)

SET 2   REPS: _____   (GOAL: 10-20 EACH SIDE)

SET 3   REPS: _____   (GOAL: 10-20 EACH SIDE)

4. PLANK

PREVIOUS BEST (WORKOUT 9)   TIME: _____

SET 1   TIME: _____   (GOAL: 45-90 SECONDS)

SET 2   TIME: _____   (GOAL: 45-90 SECONDS)

SET 3   TIME: _____   (GOAL: 45-90 SECONDS)

TODAY'S WORKOUT INTENSITY:
_____ / 10

Common Form Issue: **Chest**

Problem

You aren't squeezing your upper back together to allow your chest
to fully isolate the movement.

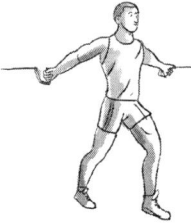

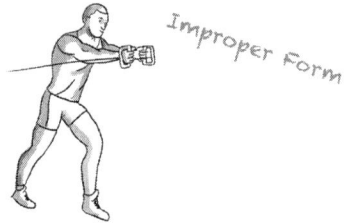

Improper Form

How to Fix This

Before performing an exercise, squeeze your upper back together very
tightly and hold it together throughout each rep.

This will minimize the support from your shoulders and triceps and allow
your chest to complete the movement. You may have to drop down in
weight significantly to do this properly.

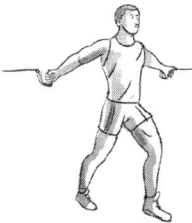

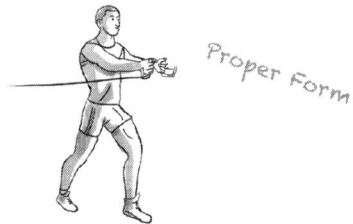

Proper Form

Exercises This Concept Applies To

All Chest Exercises!

Common Form Issue: **Biceps**

(X)

Problem

Your elbows lift upwards to help complete the movement.

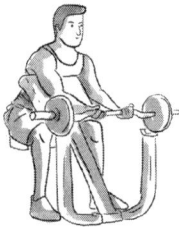

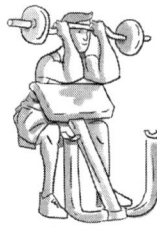

Improper Form

(✓)

How to Fix This

Your elbow should remain completely stationary during the whole movement and stay by your sides. If you can't complete the movement, go down in weight to build the proper strength first.

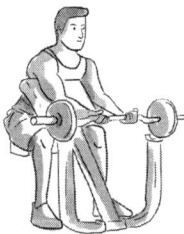

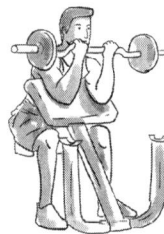

Proper Form

Exercises This Concept Applies To

All Bicep Exercises!

<u>Workout 12: Chest</u> & Biceps

DATE _____

1. FLAT BENCH PRESS

(ALTERNATIVE: FLAT BENCH DUMBBELL PRESS)

PREVIOUS BEST (WORKOUT 8)   REPS: _____   WEIGHT: _____

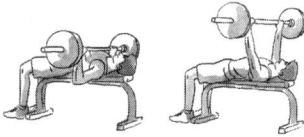

SET 1	REPS: _____	(GOAL: 10-15)	WEIGHT: _____
SET 2	REPS: _____	(GOAL: 8-12)	WEIGHT: _____
SET 3	REPS: _____	(GOAL: 6-8)	WEIGHT: _____
SET 4 (OPTIONAL)	REPS: _____	(GOAL: 4-6)	WEIGHT: _____

2. DECLINE BENCH PRESS

(ALTERNATIVE: HIGH TO LOW CABLE FLY)

PREVIOUS BEST (WORKOUT 8)   REPS: _____   WEIGHT: _____

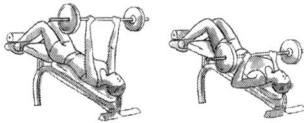

SET 1	REPS: _____	(GOAL: 10-15)	WEIGHT: _____
SET 2	REPS: _____	(GOAL: 8-12)	WEIGHT: _____
SET 3	REPS: _____	(GOAL: 6-8)	WEIGHT: _____
SET 4 (OPTIONAL)	REPS: _____	(GOAL: 4-6)	WEIGHT: _____

3. INCLINE DUMBBELL PRESS

PREVIOUS BEST (WORKOUT 8)   REPS: _____   WEIGHT: _____

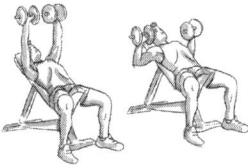

SET 1	REPS: _____	(GOAL: 10-15)	WEIGHT: _____
SET 2	REPS: _____	(GOAL: 8-12)	WEIGHT: _____
SET 3	REPS: _____	(GOAL: 6-8)	WEIGHT: _____
SET 4 (OPTIONAL)	REPS: _____	(GOAL: 4-6)	WEIGHT: _____

4. FLAT BENCH DUMBBELL FLY

(ALTERNATIVE: CHEST FLY W/ MACHINE)

PREVIOUS BEST (WORKOUT 2)   REPS: _____   WEIGHT: _____

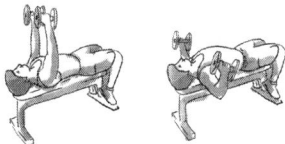

SET 1	REPS: _____	(GOAL: 10-15)	WEIGHT: _____
SET 2	REPS: _____	(GOAL: 8-12)	WEIGHT: _____
SET 3	REPS: _____	(GOAL: 6-8)	WEIGHT: _____
SET 4 (OPTIONAL)	REPS: _____	(GOAL: 4-6)	WEIGHT: _____

AMOUNT OF CARDIO DONE TODAY: _____

Workout 12: Chest & Biceps

1. PREACHER CURL
(ALTERNATIVE: SEATED DUMBBELL CURL)

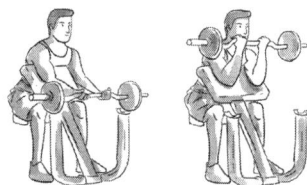

PREVIOUS BEST (WORKOUT 7)	REPS: _____		WEIGHT: _____
SET 1	REPS: _____	(GOAL: 10-15)	WEIGHT: _____
SET 2	REPS: _____	(GOAL: 8-12)	WEIGHT: _____
SET 3	REPS: _____	(GOAL: 6-8)	WEIGHT: _____
SET 4 (OPTIONAL)	REPS: _____	(GOAL: 4-6)	WEIGHT: _____

(Make sure your elbows don't move!)

2. ZOTTMAN CURL

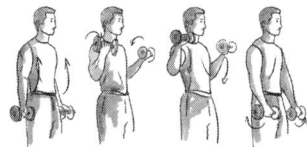

PREVIOUS BEST (WORKOUT 7)	REPS: _____		WEIGHT: _____
SET 1	REPS: _____	(GOAL: 10-15)	WEIGHT: _____
SET 2	REPS: _____	(GOAL: 8-12)	WEIGHT: _____
SET 3	REPS: _____	(GOAL: 6-8)	WEIGHT: _____
SET 4 (OPTIONAL)	REPS: _____	(GOAL: 4-6)	WEIGHT: _____

3. DUMBBELL HAMMER CURL

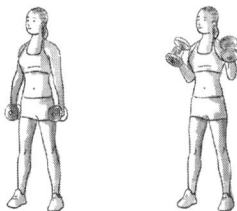

PREVIOUS BEST (WORKOUT 2)	REPS: _____		WEIGHT: _____
SET 1	REPS: _____	(GOAL: 10-15)	WEIGHT: _____
SET 2	REPS: _____	(GOAL: 8-12)	WEIGHT: _____
SET 3	REPS: _____	(GOAL: 6-8)	WEIGHT: _____
SET 4 (OPTIONAL)	REPS: _____	(GOAL: 4-6)	WEIGHT: _____

4. CONCENTRATION CURL

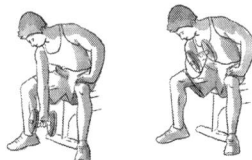

(Make sure your elbows don't move!)

PREVIOUS BEST (WORKOUT 2)	REPS: _____		WEIGHT: _____
SET 1	REPS: _____	(GOAL: 10-15)	WEIGHT: _____
SET 2	REPS: _____	(GOAL: 8-12)	WEIGHT: _____
SET 3	REPS: _____	(GOAL: 6-8)	WEIGHT: _____
SET 4 (OPTIONAL)	REPS: _____	(GOAL: 4-6)	WEIGHT: _____

TODAY'S WORKOUT INTENSITY:
_____ / 10

Workout 13: Triceps & Shoulders

DATE _____

1. SKULL CRUSHER

(Make sure to keep your wrists straight and your elbows locked in place!)

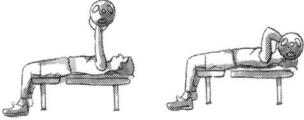

PREVIOUS BEST (WORKOUT 7) REPS: _____ WEIGHT: _____

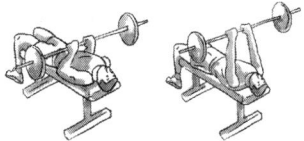

SET 1 REPS: _____ (GOAL: 10-15) WEIGHT: _____
SET 2 REPS: _____ (GOAL: 8-12) WEIGHT: _____
SET 3 REPS: _____ (GOAL: 6-8) WEIGHT: _____
SET 4 (OPTIONAL) REPS: _____ (GOAL: 4-6) WEIGHT: _____

2. CLOSE GRIP BENCH PRESS

(ALTERNATIVE: SAME MOVEMENT WITH EZ BAR) **PREVIOUS BEST** (WORKOUT 7) REPS: _____ WEIGHT: _____

SET 1 REPS: _____ (GOAL: 10-15) WEIGHT: _____
SET 2 REPS: _____ (GOAL: 8-12) WEIGHT: _____
SET 3 REPS: _____ (GOAL: 6-8) WEIGHT: _____
SET 4 (OPTIONAL) REPS: _____ (GOAL: 4-6) WEIGHT: _____

3. DIAMOND PUSH-UP

(ALTERNATIVE: ASSISTED DIP OR SEATED DIP W/ MACHINE)

(If you have trouble, you can do this on your knees.)

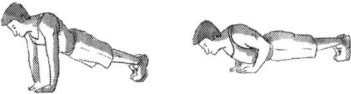

SET 1 REPS: _____ (GOAL: TO FAILURE)
SET 2 REPS: _____ (GOAL: TO FAILURE)
SET 3 REPS: _____ (GOAL: TO FAILURE)
SET 4 (OPTIONAL) REPS: _____ (GOAL: TO FAILURE)

4. ROPE PULLDOWN

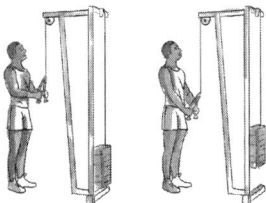

PREVIOUS BEST (WORKOUT 7) REPS: _____ WEIGHT: _____

SET 1 REPS: _____ (GOAL: 10-15) WEIGHT: _____
SET 2 REPS: _____ (GOAL: 8-12) WEIGHT: _____
SET 3 REPS: _____ (GOAL: 6-8) WEIGHT: _____
SET 4 (OPTIONAL) REPS: _____ (GOAL: 4-6) WEIGHT: _____

AMOUNT OF CARDIO DONE TODAY: _____

Workout 13: Triceps & Shoulders

1. SEATED DUMBBELL PRESS

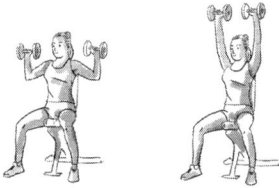

(Make sure you don't let the weights cave in towards your face, hold them straight!)

PREVIOUS BEST [WORKOUT 4]   REPS: _____   WEIGHT: _____

SET 1   REPS: _____   (GOAL: 10-15)   WEIGHT: _____
SET 2   REPS: _____   (GOAL: 8-12)   WEIGHT: _____
SET 3   REPS: _____   (GOAL: 6-8)   WEIGHT: _____
SET 4 [OPTIONAL]   REPS: _____   (GOAL: 4-6)   WEIGHT: _____

2. LATERAL DUMBBELL RAISE

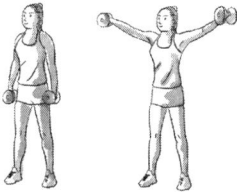

(Try not to swing your arms throughout the movement.)

PREVIOUS BEST [WORKOUT 6]   REPS: _____   WEIGHT: _____

SET 1   REPS: _____   (GOAL: 10-15)   WEIGHT: _____
SET 2   REPS: _____   (GOAL: 8-12)   WEIGHT: _____
SET 3   REPS: _____   (GOAL: 6-8)   WEIGHT: _____
SET 4 [OPTIONAL]   REPS: _____   (GOAL: 4-6)   WEIGHT: _____

3. FRONT DUMBBELL RAISE

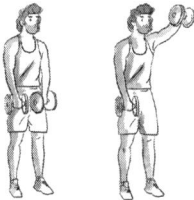

PREVIOUS BEST [WORKOUT 6]   REPS: _____   WEIGHT: _____

SET 1   REPS: _____   (GOAL: 10-15)   WEIGHT: _____
SET 2   REPS: _____   (GOAL: 8-12)   WEIGHT: _____
SET 3   REPS: _____   (GOAL: 6-8)   WEIGHT: _____
SET 4 [OPTIONAL]   REPS: _____   (GOAL: 4-6)   WEIGHT: _____

4. BARBELL RAISE

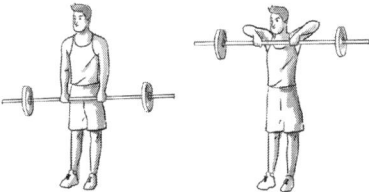

(Make sure to pull straight up and down.)

SET 1   REPS: _____   (GOAL: 10-15)   WEIGHT: _____
SET 2   REPS: _____   (GOAL: 8-12)   WEIGHT: _____
SET 3   REPS: _____   (GOAL: 6-8)   WEIGHT: _____
SET 4 [OPTIONAL]   REPS: _____   (GOAL: 4-6)   WEIGHT: _____

TODAY'S WORKOUT INTENSITY:
_____ / 10

Problem

You're skipping legs day.

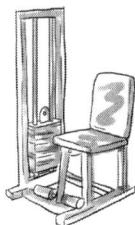

How to Fix This

Understand that legs day will drastically boost your testosterone and help fuel muscle growth for other muscles.

Also, you can lift very heavy on legs + see more drastic strength gains. These can both serve as a good confidence boost and signal that you're moving in the right direction with your training.

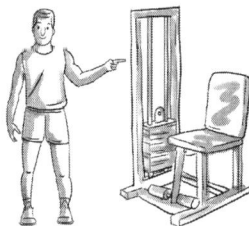

What This Concept Applies To

Getting your butt into the gym.

TODAY'S WORKOUT INTENSITY:

_____ / 10

Common Issue: **Abs**

Problem

(X)

You're overly relying on ab exercises to get visible abs.

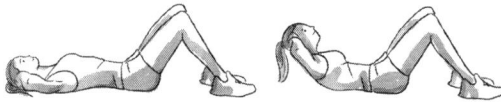

How to Fix This

(✓)

Strengthening your abs, obliques, and core has its benefits (e.g. improving posture, allowing you to lift more in other movements, etc.) but is not enough alone to visibly define your abs.

The main determinate of visible ads is going to be a low body fat % (10% or below for males, 15-20% or below for females).

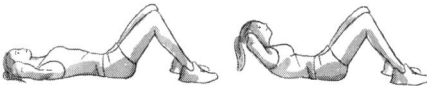

CALORIES IN   CALORIES OUT

1800 CALORIES   2300 CALORIES

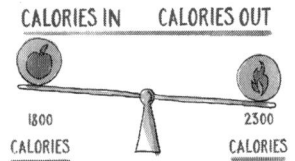

What This Concept Applies To

Improving Your Nutrition!

83

Workout 14: Legs & Abs

1. LEG PRESS
(ALTERNATIVE: DEADLIFT)

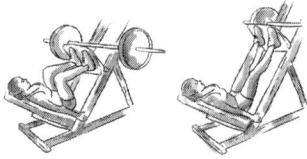

PREVIOUS BEST
(WORKOUT 3)

REPS: _____   WEIGHT: _____

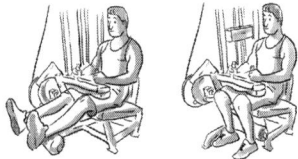

SET 1 REPS: _____ (GOAL: 10-15) WEIGHT: _____

SET 2 REPS: _____ (GOAL: 8-12) WEIGHT: _____

SET 3 REPS: _____ (GOAL: 6-8) WEIGHT: _____

SET 4 REPS: _____ (GOAL: 4-6) WEIGHT: _____
(OPTIONAL)

(Reminder: If you feel pain with any exercise, STOP!
Do NOT push through. Try a different exercise instead.)

2. HACK SQUAT
(ALTERNATIVE: BARBELL SQUAT)

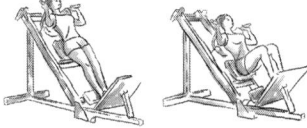

PREVIOUS BEST
(WORKOUT 3)

REPS: _____   WEIGHT: _____

SET 1 REPS: _____ (GOAL: 10-15) WEIGHT: _____

SET 2 REPS: _____ (GOAL: 8-12) WEIGHT: _____

SET 3 REPS: _____ (GOAL: 6-8) WEIGHT: _____

SET 4 REPS: _____ (GOAL: 4-6) WEIGHT: _____
(OPTIONAL)

3. WEIGHTED LUNGE
(ALTERNATIVE: QUAD EXTENSION)

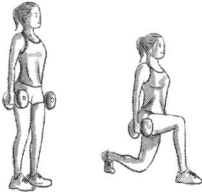

(Make sure your knees don't pass your toes when the step
is taken! The goal is to go as straight down as possible.)

SET 1 REPS: _____ (GOAL: 10-15) WEIGHT: _____

SET 2 REPS: _____ (GOAL: 8-12) WEIGHT: _____

SET 3 REPS: _____ (GOAL: 6-8) WEIGHT: _____

SET 4 REPS: _____ (GOAL: 4-6) WEIGHT: _____
(OPTIONAL)

4. HAMSTRING EXTENSION

PREVIOUS BEST
(WORKOUT 9)

REPS: _____   WEIGHT: _____

SET 1 REPS: _____ (GOAL: 10-15) WEIGHT: _____

SET 2 REPS: _____ (GOAL: 8-12) WEIGHT: _____

SET 3 REPS: _____ (GOAL: 6-8) WEIGHT: _____

SET 4 REPS: _____ (GOAL: 4-6) WEIGHT: _____
(OPTIONAL)

AMOUNT OF CARDIO DONE TODAY:
_____

Workout 14: Legs & Abs

5. CALF RAISE

(ALTERNATIVE: SEATED CALF PRESS MACHINE)

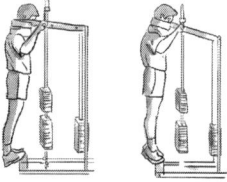

PREVIOUS BEST (WORKOUT 9)   REPS: _____   WEIGHT: _____

SET 1   REPS: _____ (GOAL: 10-15)   WEIGHT: _____

SET 2   REPS: _____ (GOAL: 8-12)   WEIGHT: _____

SET 3   REPS: _____ (GOAL: 6-8)   WEIGHT: _____

SET 4 (OPTIONAL)   REPS: _____ (GOAL: 4-6)   WEIGHT: _____

1. KNEELING CABLE CRUNCH

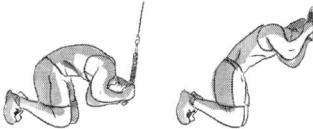

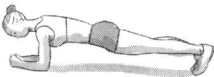

PREVIOUS BEST (WORKOUT 11)   REPS: _____   WEIGHT: _____

SET 1   REPS: _____ (GOAL: 10-20)   WEIGHT: _____

SET 2   REPS: _____ (GOAL: 10-20)   WEIGHT: _____

SET 3   REPS: _____ (GOAL: 10-20)   WEIGHT: _____

2. HANGING LEG LIFT

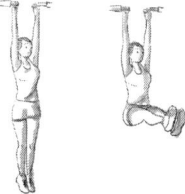

PREVIOUS BEST (WORKOUT 9)   REPS: _____

SET 1   REPS: _____ (GOAL: 10-20)

SET 2   REPS: _____ (GOAL: 10-20)

SET 3   REPS: _____ (GOAL: 10-20)

3. BICYCLE CRUNCH

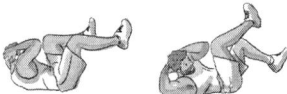

PREVIOUS BEST (WORKOUT 9)   REPS: _____

SET 1   REPS: _____ (GOAL: 10-20 EACH SIDE)

SET 2   REPS: _____ (GOAL: 10-20 EACH SIDE)

SET 3   REPS: _____ (GOAL: 10-20 EACH SIDE)

4. PLANK

PREVIOUS BEST (WORKOUT 11)   TIME: _____

SET 1   TIME: _____ (GOAL: 45-90 SECONDS)

SET 2   TIME: _____ (GOAL: 45-90 SECONDS)

SET 3   TIME: _____ (GOAL: 45-90 SECONDS)

TODAY'S WORKOUT INTENSITY:
_____ / 10

Workout 15: Full Body Circuit

DATE _____

Rest for 15-20 seconds between each exercise, then rest for 1-2 minutes after completing the entire circuit. Complete the full circuit a total of 4-5 times.

1. JUMP

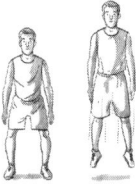

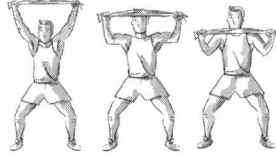

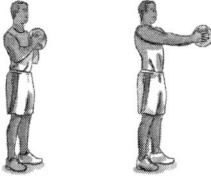

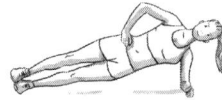

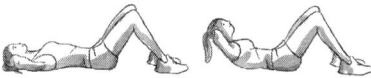

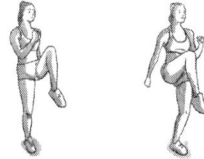

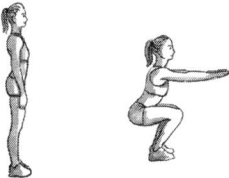

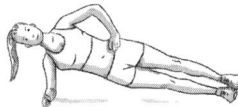

(Duration: 30 Seconds)

2. TOWEL PULL

(Duration: 30 Seconds)

3. PRAYER

(Duration: 30 Seconds)

4. SIDE PLANK

(Duration: 30 Seconds)

5. CRUNCH

(Duration: 30 Seconds)

6. HIGH KNEE

(Duration: 30 Seconds)

7. AIR SQUAT

(Duration: 30 Seconds)

8. SIDE PLANK

(Duration: 30 Seconds)

<u>Pro-Tip</u>

Push for progressive overload week after week.

You can achieve a new level of progressive overload in 3 different ways:

1. Increase the weight you use
2. Increase the reps you do, or
3. Increase the speed/intensity you complete the workout in.

You have to hit progressive overload in at least one of these ways in order to build more muscle and grow stronger.

One effective way to build this as a habit is by doing one extra rep at the end of each set once you feel you've 'really hit failure.'

If you fail and can't do that extra rep, try holding / supporting the weight for as long as possible, even if it's a half-rep (and make sure it's safe to do so without injuring yourself). This will give you a crazy additional pump.

If you DO end up completing that additional rep, that's a huge win too as you're breaking into new levels of intensity.

You'll also be learning that you may have extra fuel in the tank to push your workouts even harder. If you end up completing this extra rep, keep going to see if you can complete even more afterwards.

Aside from this method, another way to achieve progressive overload is to use a 'double progression' method.

This means that once you hit the upper range of reps for an exercise, increase the weight. Inevitably, the number of reps you can do will drop. Moving forward, stick with that new weight until you move up and exceed that rep range again.

Repeat this process as you progress through the journal.

Workout 16: Triceps & Biceps

DATE _____

1. SKULL CRUSHER

(ALTERNATIVE: CLOSE GRIP BENCH PRESS OR
OVERHEAD DUMBBELL EXTENSION)

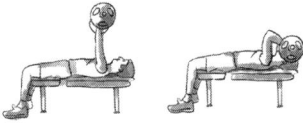

PREVIOUS BEST (WORKOUT 13)   REPS: _____ (GOAL: 4-6)   WEIGHT: _____

SET 1   REPS: _____ (GOAL: 10-15)   WEIGHT: _____

SET 2   REPS: _____ (GOAL: 8-12)   WEIGHT: _____

SET 3   REPS: _____ (GOAL: 6-8)   WEIGHT: _____

SET 4 (OPTIONAL)   REPS: _____ (GOAL: 4-6)   WEIGHT: _____

2. STRAIGHT BAR PULLDOWN

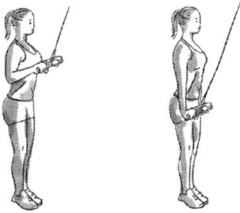

SET 1   REPS: _____ (GOAL: 10-15)   WEIGHT: _____

SET 2   REPS: _____ (GOAL: 8-12)   WEIGHT: _____

SET 3   REPS: _____ (GOAL: 6-8)   WEIGHT: _____

SET 4 (OPTIONAL)   REPS: _____ (GOAL: 4-6)   WEIGHT: _____

3. DIP

(ALTERNATIVE: ASSISTED DIP
OR SEATED DIP W/ MACHINE)

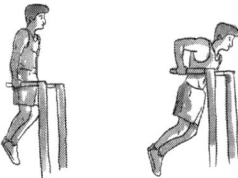

PREVIOUS BEST (WORKOUT 7)   REPS: _____   WEIGHT: _____

SET 1   REPS: _____ (GOAL: TO FAILURE)   WEIGHT: _____

SET 2   REPS: _____ (GOAL: TO FAILURE)   WEIGHT: _____

SET 3   REPS: _____ (GOAL: TO FAILURE)   WEIGHT: _____

SET 4 (OPTIONAL)   REPS: _____ (GOAL: TO FAILURE)   WEIGHT: _____

4. ROPE PULLDOWN

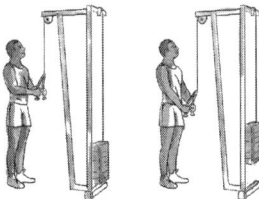

PREVIOUS BEST (WORKOUT 13)   REPS: _____   WEIGHT: _____

SET 1   REPS: _____ (GOAL: 10-15)   WEIGHT: _____

SET 2   REPS: _____ (GOAL: 8-12)   WEIGHT: _____

SET 3   REPS: _____ (GOAL: 6-8)   WEIGHT: _____

SET 4 (OPTIONAL)   REPS: _____ (GOAL: 4-6)   WEIGHT: _____

🏃 **AMOUNT OF CARDIO DONE TODAY:**
_____

Workout 16: Triceps & Biceps

1. CONCENTRATION CURL

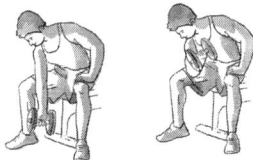

PREVIOUS BEST
(WORKOUT 12)   REPS: _____   WEIGHT: _____

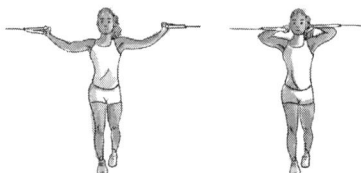

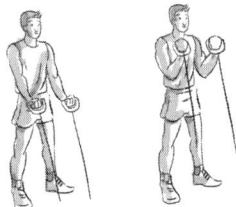

SET 1   REPS: _____   (GOAL: 10-15)   WEIGHT: _____

SET 2   REPS: _____   (GOAL: 8-12)   WEIGHT: _____

SET 3   REPS: _____   (GOAL: 6-8)   WEIGHT: _____

SET 4   REPS: _____   (GOAL: 4-6)   WEIGHT: _____
(OPTIONAL)

2. ROPE HAMMER CURL

(ALTERNATIVE: SEATED HAMMER CURL)

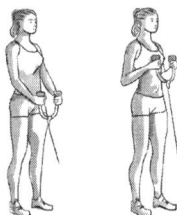

PREVIOUS BEST
(WORKOUT 7)   REPS: _____   WEIGHT: _____

SET 1   REPS: _____   (GOAL: 10-15)   WEIGHT: _____

SET 2   REPS: _____   (GOAL: 8-12)   WEIGHT: _____

SET 3   REPS: _____   (GOAL: 6-8)   WEIGHT: _____

SET 4   REPS: _____   (GOAL: 4-6)   WEIGHT: _____
(OPTIONAL)

3. OVERHEAD CABLE CURL

PREVIOUS BEST
(WORKOUT 2)   REPS: _____   WEIGHT: _____

SET 1   REPS: _____   (GOAL: 10-15)   WEIGHT: _____

SET 2   REPS: _____   (GOAL: 8-12)   WEIGHT: _____

SET 3   REPS: _____   (GOAL: 6-8)   WEIGHT: _____

SET 4   REPS: _____   (GOAL: 4-6)   WEIGHT: _____
(OPTIONAL)

4. UNDERHAND CABLE CURL

PREVIOUS BEST
(WORKOUT 7)   REPS: _____   WEIGHT: _____

SET 1   REPS: _____   (GOAL: 10-15)   WEIGHT: _____

SET 2   REPS: _____   (GOAL: 8-12)   WEIGHT: _____

SET 3   REPS: _____   (GOAL: 6-8)   WEIGHT: _____

SET 4   REPS: _____   (GOAL: 4-6)   WEIGHT: _____
(OPTIONAL)

TODAY'S WORKOUT INTENSITY:

_____ / 10

Workout 17: Chest & Abs

DATE _____

1. FLAT BENCH PRESS

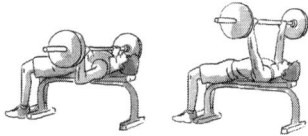

PREVIOUS BEST (WORKOUT 12) REPS: _____ WEIGHT: _____

SET 1 REPS: _____ (GOAL: 10-15) WEIGHT: _____
SET 2 REPS: _____ (GOAL: 8-12) WEIGHT: _____
SET 3 REPS: _____ (GOAL: 6-8) WEIGHT: _____
SET 4 (OPTIONAL) REPS: _____ (GOAL: 4-6) WEIGHT: _____

2. DECLINE BENCH PRESS

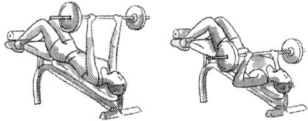

PREVIOUS BEST (WORKOUT 12) REPS: _____ WEIGHT: _____

SET 1 REPS: _____ (GOAL: 10-15) WEIGHT: _____
SET 2 REPS: _____ (GOAL: 8-12) WEIGHT: _____
SET 3 REPS: _____ (GOAL: 6-8) WEIGHT: _____
SET 4 (OPTIONAL) REPS: _____ (GOAL: 4-6) WEIGHT: _____

3. INCLINE DUMBBELL FLY

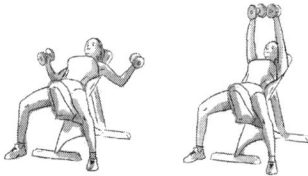

PREVIOUS BEST (WORKOUT 8) REPS: _____ WEIGHT: _____

SET 1 REPS: _____ (GOAL: 10-15) WEIGHT: _____
SET 2 REPS: _____ (GOAL: 8-12) WEIGHT: _____
SET 3 REPS: _____ (GOAL: 6-8) WEIGHT: _____
SET 4 (OPTIONAL) REPS: _____ (GOAL: 4-6) WEIGHT: _____

4. DUMBBELL PULLOVER

(Make sure you stop the movement when the dumbbell comes over your chest and squeeze tightly.)

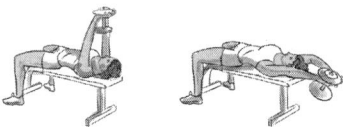

SET 1 REPS: _____ (GOAL: 10-15) WEIGHT: _____
SET 2 REPS: _____ (GOAL: 8-12) WEIGHT: _____
SET 3 REPS: _____ (GOAL: 6-8) WEIGHT: _____
SET 4 (OPTIONAL) REPS: _____ (GOAL: 4-6) WEIGHT: _____

AMOUNT OF CARDIO DONE TODAY: _____

90

Workout 17: Chest & Abs

5. CABLE CROSSOVER

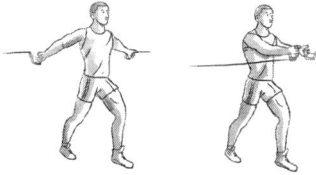

	PREVIOUS BEST (WORKOUT 3)	REPS: _____		WEIGHT: _____
	SET 1	REPS: _____	(GOAL: 10-15)	WEIGHT: _____
	SET 2	REPS: _____	(GOAL: 8-12)	WEIGHT: _____
	SET 3	REPS: _____	(GOAL: 6-8)	WEIGHT: _____
	SET 4 (OPTIONAL)	REPS: _____	(GOAL: 4-6)	WEIGHT: _____

1. KNEELING CABLE CRUNCH

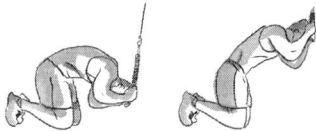

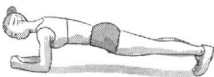

	PREVIOUS BEST (WORKOUT 14)	REPS: _____		WEIGHT: _____
	SET 1	REPS: _____	(GOAL: 10-20)	WEIGHT: _____
	SET 2	REPS: _____	(GOAL: 10-20)	WEIGHT: _____
	SET 3	REPS: _____	(GOAL: 10-20)	WEIGHT: _____

2. LEG LIFT

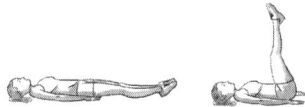

	PREVIOUS BEST (WORKOUT 11)	REPS: _____	
	SET 1	REPS: _____	(GOAL: 10-20)
	SET 2	REPS: _____	(GOAL: 10-20)
	SET 3	REPS: _____	(GOAL: 10-20)

3. STARFISH CRUNCH

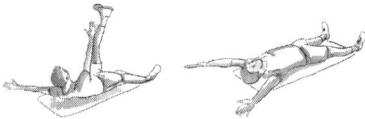

	PREVIOUS BEST (WORKOUT 3)	REPS: _____	
	SET 1	REPS: _____	(GOAL: 10-20 EACH SIDE)
	SET 2	REPS: _____	(GOAL: 10-20 EACH SIDE)
	SET 3	REPS: _____	(GOAL: 10-20 EACH SIDE)

4. PLANK

	PREVIOUS BEST (WORKOUT 14)	TIME: _____	
	SET 1	TIME: _____	(GOAL: 45-90 SECONDS)
	SET 2	TIME: _____	(GOAL: 45-90 SECONDS)
	SET 3	TIME: _____	(GOAL: 45-90 SECONDS)

TODAY'S WORKOUT INTENSITY:
_____ / 10

Common Form Issue: **Back**

Problem

After completing a rep, you aren't allowing your lats to fully extend when releasing the movement back towards the starting position.

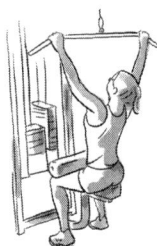

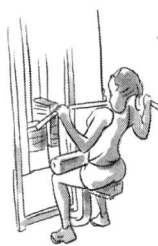

Improper Form

How to Fix This

Allow your lats to fully relax and stretch out back towards the starting position. Make sure to still maintain control of the weight as you return it to that stretched position. When beginning the next rep, use your lats (not your arms) to move the weights again.

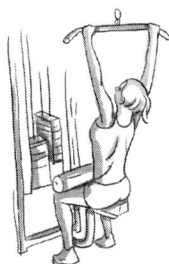

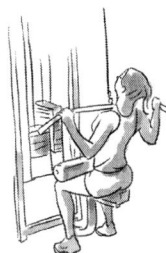

Proper Form

Exercises This Concept Applies To

Bent Over Dumbbell Row, Close Grip Cable Row, Reverse Grip Lat Pulldown, T-Bar Row

Common Form Issue: **Shoulders**

(X) ***Problem***

You're overly using your traps throughout the movement.

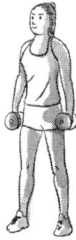

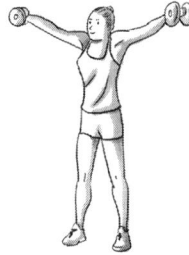

Improper Form

(✓) ***How to Fix This***

Allow your traps to fall downwards and fully disengage, isolating as much of your shoulder muscles as possible to complete the movement.

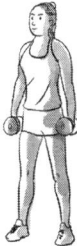

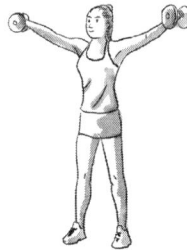

Proper Form

Exercises This Concept Applies To

All Shoulders Exercises (Except Shrugs)!

Workout 18: Back & Shoulders

DATE _____

1. CLOSE GRIP CABLE ROW

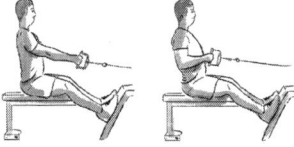

PREVIOUS BEST
(WORKOUT 11)

REPS: _____

WEIGHT: _____

SET 1 REPS: _____ (GOAL: 10-15) WEIGHT: _____

SET 2 REPS: _____ (GOAL: 8-12) WEIGHT: _____

SET 3 REPS: _____ (GOAL: 6-8) WEIGHT: _____

SET 4 REPS: _____ (GOAL: 4-6) WEIGHT: _____
[OPTIONAL]

2. T-BAR ROW

(ALTERNATIVE: BENT OVER DUMBBELL ROW)

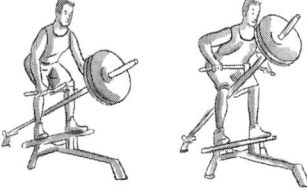

PREVIOUS BEST
(WORKOUT 11)

REPS: _____

WEIGHT: _____

SET 1 REPS: _____ (GOAL: 10-15) WEIGHT: _____

SET 2 REPS: _____ (GOAL: 8-12) WEIGHT: _____

SET 3 REPS: _____ (GOAL: 6-8) WEIGHT: _____

SET 4 REPS: _____ (GOAL: 4-6) WEIGHT: _____
[OPTIONAL]

3. LAT PULLDOWN

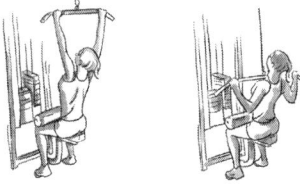

(Make sure to move faster on the pull and slower on the way up to feel the resistance.)

PREVIOUS BEST
(WORKOUT 6)

REPS: _____

WEIGHT: _____

SET 1 REPS: _____ (GOAL: 10-15) WEIGHT: _____

SET 2 REPS: _____ (GOAL: 8-12) WEIGHT: _____

SET 3 REPS: _____ (GOAL: 6-8) WEIGHT: _____

SET 4 REPS: _____ (GOAL: 4-6) WEIGHT: _____
[OPTIONAL]

4. STRAIGHT ARM PULLDOWN

(ALTERNATIVE: PULL-UP)

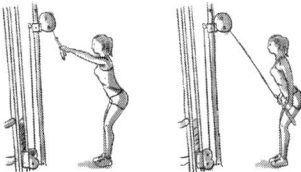

PREVIOUS BEST
(WORKOUT 11)

REPS: _____

WEIGHT: _____

SET 1 REPS: _____ (GOAL: 10-15) WEIGHT: _____

SET 2 REPS: _____ (GOAL: 8-12) WEIGHT: _____

SET 3 REPS: _____ (GOAL: 6-8) WEIGHT: _____

SET 4 REPS: _____ (GOAL: 4-6) WEIGHT: _____
[OPTIONAL]

AMOUNT OF CARDIO DONE TODAY:
_____

Workout 18: Back & Shoulders

1. ARNOLD DUMBBELL PRESS

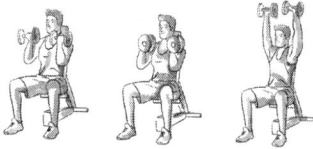

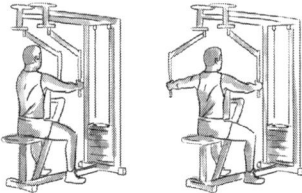

PREVIOUS BEST			
(WORKOUT 6)	REPS: _____		WEIGHT: _____
SET 1	REPS: _____	(GOAL: 10-15)	WEIGHT: _____
SET 2	REPS: _____	(GOAL: 8-12)	WEIGHT: _____
SET 3	REPS: _____	(GOAL: 6-8)	WEIGHT: _____
SET 4 (OPTIONAL)	REPS: _____	(GOAL: 4-6)	WEIGHT: _____

(You can also do this with cable handles.)

2. LATERAL DUMBBELL RAISE

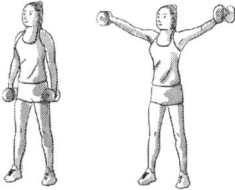

PREVIOUS BEST			
(WORKOUT 13)	REPS: _____		WEIGHT: _____
SET 1	REPS: _____	(GOAL: 10-15)	WEIGHT: _____
SET 2	REPS: _____	(GOAL: 8-12)	WEIGHT: _____
SET 3	REPS: _____	(GOAL: 6-8)	WEIGHT: _____
SET 4 (OPTIONAL)	REPS: _____	(GOAL: 4-6)	WEIGHT: _____

3. REVERSE FLY

PREVIOUS BEST			
(WORKOUT 6)	REPS: _____		WEIGHT: _____
SET 1	REPS: _____	(GOAL: 10-15)	WEIGHT: _____
SET 2	REPS: _____	(GOAL: 8-12)	WEIGHT: _____
SET 3	REPS: _____	(GOAL: 6-8)	WEIGHT: _____
SET 4 (OPTIONAL)	REPS: _____	(GOAL: 4-6)	WEIGHT: _____

4. SHRUG

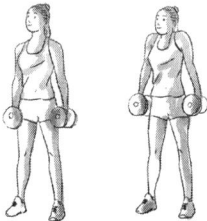

PREVIOUS BEST			
(WORKOUT 4)	REPS: _____		WEIGHT: _____
SET 1	REPS: _____	(GOAL: 10-15)	WEIGHT: _____
SET 2	REPS: _____	(GOAL: 8-12)	WEIGHT: _____
SET 3	REPS: _____	(GOAL: 6-8)	WEIGHT: _____
SET 4 (OPTIONAL)	REPS: _____	(GOAL: 4-6)	WEIGHT: _____

TODAY'S WORKOUT INTENSITY:
_____ / 10

Workout 19: Legs & Forearms

DATE _____

1. DEADLIFT

(ALTERNATIVE: LEG PRESS)

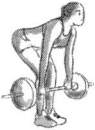

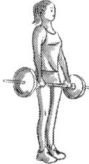

PREVIOUS BEST (WORKOUT 9)   REPS: _____   WEIGHT: _____

SET 1	REPS: _____	(GOAL: 10-15)	WEIGHT: _____
SET 2	REPS: _____	(GOAL: 8-12)	WEIGHT: _____
SET 3	REPS: _____	(GOAL: 6-8)	WEIGHT: _____
SET 4 (OPTIONAL)	REPS: _____	(GOAL: 4-6)	WEIGHT: _____

2. BARBELL SQUAT

(ALTERNATIVE: HACK SQUAT)

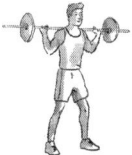

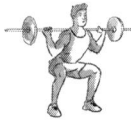

PREVIOUS BEST (WORKOUT 9)   REPS: _____   WEIGHT: _____

SET 1	REPS: _____	(GOAL: 10-15)	WEIGHT: _____
SET 2	REPS: _____	(GOAL: 8-12)	WEIGHT: _____
SET 3	REPS: _____	(GOAL: 6-8)	WEIGHT: _____
SET 4 (OPTIONAL)	REPS: _____	(GOAL: 4-6)	WEIGHT: _____

3. QUAD EXTENSION

(ALTERNATIVE: WEIGHTED LUNGE)

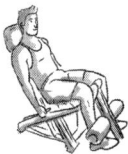

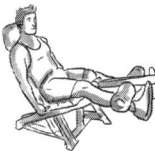

PREVIOUS BEST (WORKOUT 9)   REPS: _____   WEIGHT: _____

SET 1	REPS: _____	(GOAL: 10-15)	WEIGHT: _____
SET 2	REPS: _____	(GOAL: 8-12)	WEIGHT: _____
SET 3	REPS: _____	(GOAL: 6-8)	WEIGHT: _____
SET 4 (OPTIONAL)	REPS: _____	(GOAL: 4-6)	WEIGHT: _____

4. HAMSTRING EXTENSION

PREVIOUS BEST (WORKOUT 14)   REPS: _____   WEIGHT: _____

SET 1	REPS: _____	(GOAL: 10-15)	WEIGHT: _____
SET 2	REPS: _____	(GOAL: 8-12)	WEIGHT: _____
SET 3	REPS: _____	(GOAL: 6-8)	WEIGHT: _____
SET 4 (OPTIONAL)	REPS: _____	(GOAL: 4-6)	WEIGHT: _____

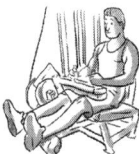

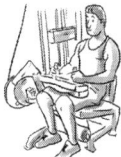

🏃 **AMOUNT OF CARDIO DONE TODAY:**
_____

Workout 19: Legs & Forearms

5. CALF RAISE

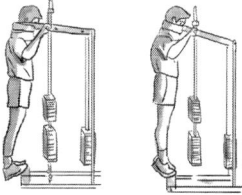

PREVIOUS BEST (WORKOUT 14)	REPS: _____		WEIGHT: _____
SET 1	REPS: _____	(GOAL: 10-15)	WEIGHT: _____
SET 2	REPS: _____	(GOAL: 8-12)	WEIGHT: _____
SET 3	REPS: _____	(GOAL: 6-8)	WEIGHT: _____
SET 4 (OPTIONAL)	REPS: _____	(GOAL: 4-6)	WEIGHT: _____

1. REVERSE GRIP DUMBBELL CURL

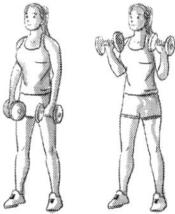

SET 1	REPS: _____	(GOAL: 10-15)	WEIGHT: _____
SET 2	REPS: _____	(GOAL: 8-12)	WEIGHT: _____
SET 3	REPS: _____	(GOAL: 6-8)	WEIGHT: _____
SET 4 (OPTIONAL)	REPS: _____	(GOAL: 4-6)	WEIGHT: _____

2. DUMBBELL TWIST-UP

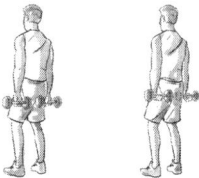

SET 1	REPS: _____	(GOAL: 10-15)	WEIGHT: _____
SET 2	REPS: _____	(GOAL: 8-12)	WEIGHT: _____
SET 3	REPS: _____	(GOAL: 6-8)	WEIGHT: _____
SET 4 (OPTIONAL)	REPS: _____	(GOAL: 4-6)	WEIGHT: _____

TODAY'S WORKOUT INTENSITY:
_____ / 10

.

Workout 20: Full Body Circuit

> Rest for *15-20 seconds* between each exercise, then rest for *1-2 minutes* after completing the entire circuit. Complete the full circuit *a total of 4-5 times.*

1. RUN IN PLACE

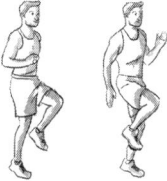

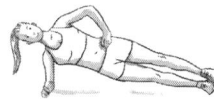

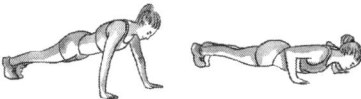

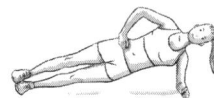

(Duration: 30 Seconds)

2. MOUNTAIN CLIMBER

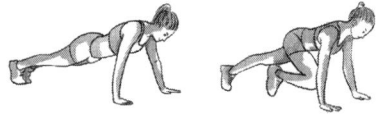

(Duration: 30 Seconds)

3. STARFISH CRUNCH

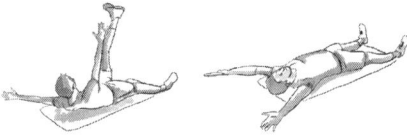

(Duration: 30 Seconds)

4. SIDE PLANK

(Duration: 30 Seconds)

5. ALTERNATING LUNGE

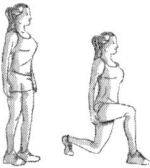

(Duration: 30 Seconds)

6. TOWEL SNATCH

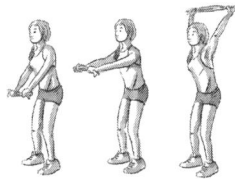

(Duration: 30 Seconds)

7. PUSH-UP

(Duration: 30 Seconds)

8. SIDE PLANK

(Duration: 30 Seconds)

TODAY'S WORKOUT INTENSITY:
_____ / 10

<u>Check-In</u>

How am I feeling about the quality and intensity of my last 10 workouts compared to the first 10 workouts?

_____

_____

_____

_____

What changes am I noticing in my body?

_____

_____

_____

_____

When I'm working out, what takes my attention from the gym and being fully engaged mentally in my workouts?

_____

_____

_____

_____

Am I beginning to see how much I can change if I stick to this program?

_____

_____

_____

_____

Bonus Challenge

> *Going forward, add in two supersets (four exercises) in each workout.*

This is the first optional challenge presented in this journal.

Taking this on would mean that in each workout, you would perform two exercises back-to-back. You would do this twice in each workout, supersetting a total of four exercises.

Supersets work as follows: for the two exercises you're working on, you would complete set one of each back-to-back without any rest. You rest only after finishing both, then repeat with their remaining sets. You superset 1 exercise for one muscle with 1 exercise for the other muscle being worked that day.

Supersets don't necessarily have to be done in the same order the exercises are listed on each page. To minimize unnecessary walking time / losing machines, try to superset exercises that are near each other in your gym.

One large benefit of supersets is they **vastly** speed up your workout completion time.

Experiment with it and choose what will work best for you / your gym.

_____

(Optional)
I will complete two supersets (four exercises) each workout for the next week.

_____   _____

Signature   Date

Workout 21: Back & Abs

DATE _____

(Unlike all other exercises, the HIGHER the weight used on assisted pull-ups and assisted dips, the EASIER the exercise is.)

1. ASSISTED PULL-UP
(ALTERNATIVE: PULL-UP OR TOWEL PULL)

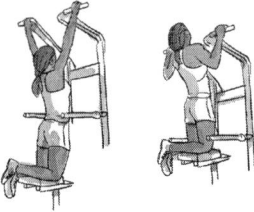

PREVIOUS BEST
(WORKOUT 11)

REPS: _____   WEIGHT: _____

SET 1   REPS: _____ (GOAL: 10-15)   WEIGHT: _____

SET 2   REPS: _____ (GOAL: 8-12)   WEIGHT: _____

SET 3   REPS: _____ (GOAL: 6-8)   WEIGHT: _____

SET 4   REPS: _____ (GOAL: 4-6)   WEIGHT: _____
(OPTIONAL)

2. BENT OVER DUMBBELL ROW

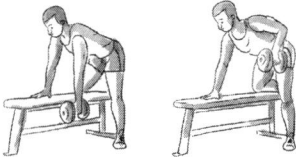

PREVIOUS BEST
(WORKOUT 6)

REPS: _____   WEIGHT: _____

SET 1   REPS: _____ (GOAL: 10-15)   WEIGHT: _____

SET 2   REPS: _____ (GOAL: 8-12)   WEIGHT: _____

SET 3   REPS: _____ (GOAL: 6-8)   WEIGHT: _____

SET 4   REPS: _____ (GOAL: 4-6)   WEIGHT: _____
(OPTIONAL)

3. STRAIGHT ARM PULLDOWN

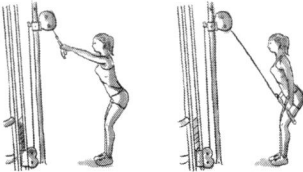

PREVIOUS BEST
(WORKOUT 18)

REPS: _____   WEIGHT: _____

SET 1   REPS: _____ (GOAL: 10-15)   WEIGHT: _____

SET 2   REPS: _____ (GOAL: 8-12)   WEIGHT: _____

SET 3   REPS: _____ (GOAL: 6-8)   WEIGHT: _____

SET 4   REPS: _____ (GOAL: 4-6)   WEIGHT: _____
(OPTIONAL)

4. REVERSE GRIP LAT PULLDOWN

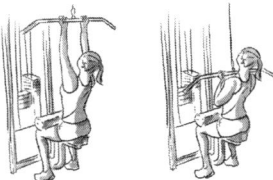

PREVIOUS BEST
(WORKOUT 11)

REPS: _____   WEIGHT: _____

SET 1   REPS: _____ (GOAL: 10-15)   WEIGHT: _____

SET 2   REPS: _____ (GOAL: 8-12)   WEIGHT: _____

SET 3   REPS: _____ (GOAL: 6-8)   WEIGHT: _____

SET 4   REPS: _____ (GOAL: 4-6)   WEIGHT: _____
(OPTIONAL)

AMOUNT OF CARDIO DONE TODAY:
_____

Workout 21: Back & Abs

5. UPPER BACK ROPE PULL

(This also works the rear part of your shoulder.)

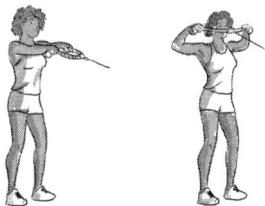

SET 1	REPS: _____ (GOAL: 10-15)	WEIGHT: _____
SET 2	REPS: _____ (GOAL: 8-12)	WEIGHT: _____
SET 3	REPS: _____ (GOAL: 6-8)	WEIGHT: _____
SET 4 (OPTIONAL)	REPS: _____ (GOAL: 4-6)	WEIGHT: _____

1. KNEELING CABLE CRUNCH

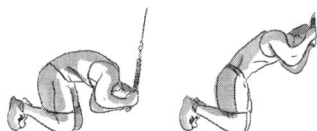

PREVIOUS BEST (WORKOUT 17)   REPS: _____   WEIGHT: _____

SET 1	REPS: _____ (GOAL: 10-20)	WEIGHT: _____
SET 2	REPS: _____ (GOAL: 10-20)	WEIGHT: _____
SET 3	REPS: _____ (GOAL: 10-20)	WEIGHT: _____

2. RUSSIAN TWIST

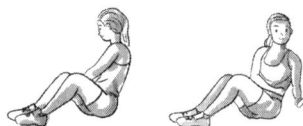

PREVIOUS BEST (WORKOUT 11)   REPS: _____

SET 1	REPS: _____ (GOAL: 10-20 EACH SIDE)
SET 2	REPS: _____ (GOAL: 10-20 EACH SIDE)
SET 3	REPS: _____ (GOAL: 10-20 EACH SIDE)

3. STARFISH CRUNCH

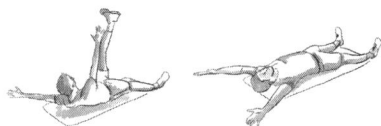

PREVIOUS BEST (WORKOUT 17)   REPS: _____

SET 1	REPS: _____ (GOAL: 10-20 EACH SIDE)
SET 2	REPS: _____ (GOAL: 10-20 EACH SIDE)
SET 3	REPS: _____ (GOAL: 10-20 EACH SIDE)

4. BICYCLE CRUNCH

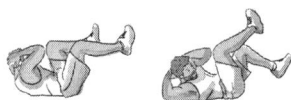

PREVIOUS BEST (WORKOUT 14)   TIME: _____

SET 1	REPS: _____ (GOAL: 10-20 EACH SIDE)
SET 2	REPS: _____ (GOAL: 10-20 EACH SIDE)
SET 3	REPS: _____ (GOAL: 10-20 EACH SIDE)

SUPERSETS DONE TODAY (CIRCLE):
1   2   3   4

TODAY'S WORKOUT INTENSITY:
_____ / 10

Problem

Your traps are bunched up and shoulders aren't dropped down.

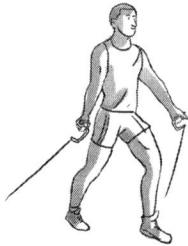

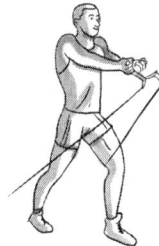

Improper Form

How to Fix This

Allow your traps and shoulders to drop fully during the movement to use them as little as possible. You want to disengage them and let them relax, allowing your chest to carry the majority of the weight during the movement.

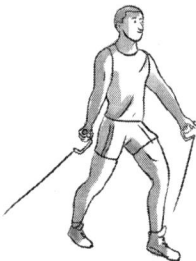

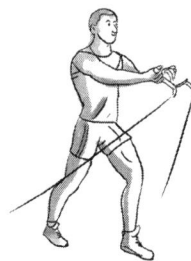

Proper Form

Exercises This Concept Applies To

All Cable & Machine Flies!

Common Form Issue: **Biceps**

(X)

Problem

Your wrists bend during the movement.

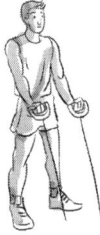

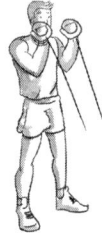

Improper Form

(✓)

How to Fix This

Similar to maintaining proper form with your triceps, Imagine a metal rod is going through your arm, your wrist, and up to your fingers. Don't allow any bending to occur throughout the movement. This will likely lead to more use of your finger strength (grip) and more forearm strength.

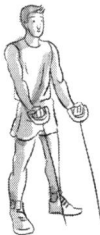

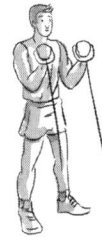

Proper Form

Exercises This Concept Applies To

All Bicep Exercises!

Workout 22: Chest & Biceps

1. FLAT BENCH PRESS

(ALTERNATIVE: FLAT BENCH DUMBBELL PRESS)

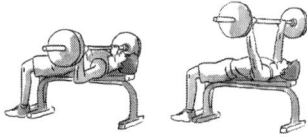

PREVIOUS BEST
(WORKOUT 17)

REPS: _____   WEIGHT: _____

SET 1   REPS: _____   (GOAL: 10-15)   WEIGHT: _____

SET 2   REPS: _____   (GOAL: 8-12)   WEIGHT: _____

SET 3   REPS: _____   (GOAL: 6-8)   WEIGHT: _____

SET 4   REPS: _____   (GOAL: 4-6)   WEIGHT: _____
(OPTIONAL)

2. HIGH TO LOW CABLE FLY

(Try putting one leg forward for balance.)

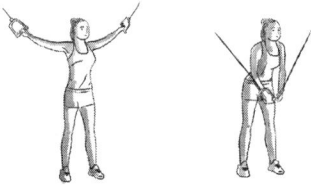

SET 1   REPS: _____   (GOAL: 10-15)   WEIGHT: _____

SET 2   REPS: _____   (GOAL: 8-12)   WEIGHT: _____

SET 3   REPS: _____   (GOAL: 6-8)   WEIGHT: _____

SET 4   REPS: _____   (GOAL: 4-6)   WEIGHT: _____
(OPTIONAL)

3. LOW TO HIGH CABLE FLY

(Make sure to keep your arms as straight as
possible to prevent yourself from using your bicep.)

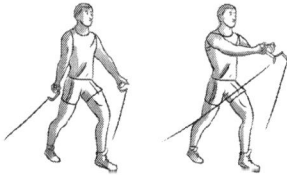

SET 1   REPS: _____   (GOAL: 10-15)   WEIGHT: _____

SET 2   REPS: _____   (GOAL: 8-12)   WEIGHT: _____

SET 3   REPS: _____   (GOAL: 6-8)   WEIGHT: _____

SET 4   REPS: _____   (GOAL: 4-6)   WEIGHT: _____
(OPTIONAL)

4. CABLE FLY

(ALTERNATIVE: CHEST FLY W/ MACHINE)

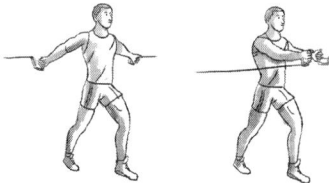

SET 1   REPS: _____   (GOAL: 10-15)   WEIGHT: _____

SET 2   REPS: _____   (GOAL: 8-12)   WEIGHT: _____

SET 3   REPS: _____   (GOAL: 6-8)   WEIGHT: _____

SET 4   REPS: _____   (GOAL: 4-6)   WEIGHT: _____
(OPTIONAL)

🏃 **AMOUNT OF CARDIO DONE TODAY:**
_____

Workout 22: Chest & Biceps

1. PREACHER CURL

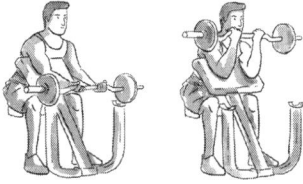

PREVIOUS BEST (WORKOUT 12)	REPS: _____		WEIGHT: _____
SET 1	REPS: _____	(GOAL: 10-15)	WEIGHT: _____
SET 2	REPS: _____	(GOAL: 8-12)	WEIGHT: _____
SET 3	REPS: _____	(GOAL: 6-8)	WEIGHT: _____
SET 4 (OPTIONAL)	REPS: _____	(GOAL: 4-6)	WEIGHT: _____

2. DUMBBELL HAMMER CURL

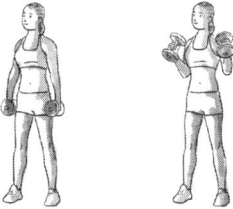

PREVIOUS BEST (WORKOUT 12)	REPS: _____		WEIGHT: _____
SET 1	REPS: _____	(GOAL: 10-15)	WEIGHT: _____
SET 2	REPS: _____	(GOAL: 8-12)	WEIGHT: _____
SET 3	REPS: _____	(GOAL: 6-8)	WEIGHT: _____
SET 4 (OPTIONAL)	REPS: _____	(GOAL: 4-6)	WEIGHT: _____

3. OVERHEAD CABLE CURL

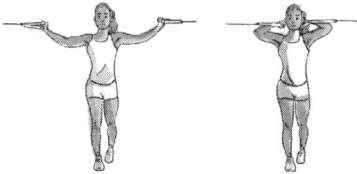

PREVIOUS BEST (WORKOUT 16)	REPS: _____		WEIGHT: _____
SET 1	REPS: _____	(GOAL: 10-15)	WEIGHT: _____
SET 2	REPS: _____	(GOAL: 8-12)	WEIGHT: _____
SET 3	REPS: _____	(GOAL: 6-8)	WEIGHT: _____
SET 4 (OPTIONAL)	REPS: _____	(GOAL: 4-6)	WEIGHT: _____

4. ROPE HAMMER CURL

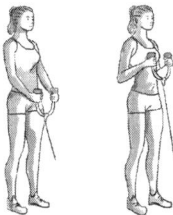

PREVIOUS BEST (WORKOUT 16)	REPS: _____		WEIGHT: _____
SET 1	REPS: _____	(GOAL: 10-15)	WEIGHT: _____
SET 2	REPS: _____	(GOAL: 8-12)	WEIGHT: _____
SET 3	REPS: _____	(GOAL: 6-8)	WEIGHT: _____
SET 4 (OPTIONAL)	REPS: _____	(GOAL: 4-6)	WEIGHT: _____

SUPERSETS DONE TODAY (CIRCLE):

1   2   3   4

TODAY'S WORKOUT INTENSITY:

_____ / 10

EXERCISE
GUIDE

Workout 23: Shoulders & Triceps

DATE

1. LATERAL DUMBBELL RAISE

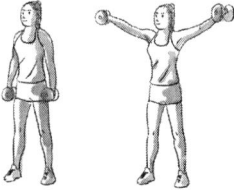

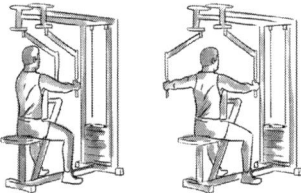

PREVIOUS BEST (WORKOUT 18)	REPS: _____	WEIGHT: _____
SET 1	REPS: _____ (GOAL: 10-15)	WEIGHT: _____
SET 2	REPS: _____ (GOAL: 8-12)	WEIGHT: _____
SET 3	REPS: _____ (GOAL: 6-8)	WEIGHT: _____
SET 4 (OPTIONAL)	REPS: _____ (GOAL: 4-6)	WEIGHT: _____

2. BARBELL RAISE

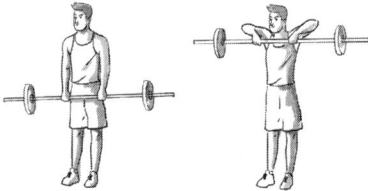

PREVIOUS BEST (WORKOUT 13)	REPS: _____	WEIGHT: _____
SET 1	REPS: _____ (GOAL: 10-15)	WEIGHT: _____
SET 2	REPS: _____ (GOAL: 8-12)	WEIGHT: _____
SET 3	REPS: _____ (GOAL: 6-8)	WEIGHT: _____
SET 4 (OPTIONAL)	REPS: _____ (GOAL: 4-6)	WEIGHT: _____

3. REVERSE FLY

PREVIOUS BEST (WORKOUT 18)	REPS: _____	WEIGHT: _____
SET 1	REPS: _____ (GOAL: 10-15)	WEIGHT: _____
SET 2	REPS: _____ (GOAL: 8-12)	WEIGHT: _____
SET 3	REPS: _____ (GOAL: 6-8)	WEIGHT: _____
SET 4 (OPTIONAL)	REPS: _____ (GOAL: 4-6)	WEIGHT: _____

4. SEATED DUMBBELL PRESS

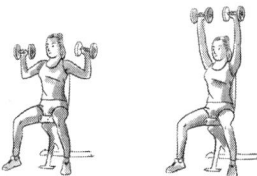

PREVIOUS BEST (WORKOUT 13)	REPS: _____	WEIGHT: _____
SET 1	REPS: _____ (GOAL: 10-15)	WEIGHT: _____
SET 2	REPS: _____ (GOAL: 8-12)	WEIGHT: _____
SET 3	REPS: _____ (GOAL: 6-8)	WEIGHT: _____
SET 4 (OPTIONAL)	REPS: _____ (GOAL: 4-6)	WEIGHT: _____

AMOUNT OF CARDIO DONE TODAY:

....

Workout 23: Shoulders & Triceps

1. SKULL CRUSHER

(ALTERNATIVE: CLOSE GRIP BENCH PRESS OR
DUMBBELL PULLOVER)

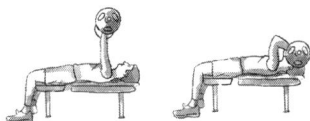

PREVIOUS BEST
(WORKOUT 16)

REPS: _____   WEIGHT: _____

SET 1   REPS: _____ (GOAL: 10-15)   WEIGHT: _____
SET 2   REPS: _____ (GOAL: 8-12)   WEIGHT: _____
SET 3   REPS: _____ (GOAL: 6-8)   WEIGHT: _____
SET 4   REPS: _____ (GOAL: 4-6)   WEIGHT: _____
(OPTIONAL)

(Keep your elbows in place throughout the whole exercise so they don't move!)

2. OVERHEAD DUMBBELL EXTENSION

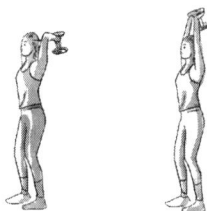

PREVIOUS BEST
(WORKOUT 1)

REPS: _____   WEIGHT: _____

SET 1   REPS: _____ (GOAL: 10-15)   WEIGHT: _____
SET 2   REPS: _____ (GOAL: 8-12)   WEIGHT: _____
SET 3   REPS: _____ (GOAL: 6-8)   WEIGHT: _____
SET 4   REPS: _____ (GOAL: 4-6)   WEIGHT: _____
(OPTIONAL)

3. ROPE PULLDOWN

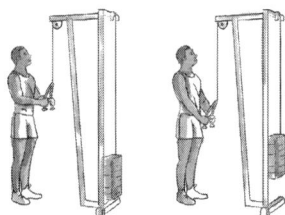

PREVIOUS BEST
(WORKOUT 16)

REPS: _____   WEIGHT: _____

SET 1   REPS: _____ (GOAL: 10-15)   WEIGHT: _____
SET 2   REPS: _____ (GOAL: 8-12)   WEIGHT: _____
SET 3   REPS: _____ (GOAL: 6-8)   WEIGHT: _____
SET 4   REPS: _____ (GOAL: 4-6)   WEIGHT: _____
(OPTIONAL)

4. DIP

(ALTERNATIVE: ASSISTED DIP
OR SEATED DIP W/ MACHINE)

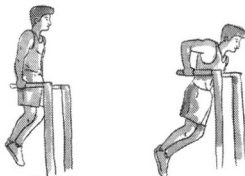

PREVIOUS BEST
(WORKOUT 16)

REPS: _____   WEIGHT: _____

SET 1   REPS: _____ (GOAL: TO FAILURE)   WEIGHT: _____
SET 2   REPS: _____ (GOAL: TO FAILURE)   WEIGHT: _____
SET 3   REPS: _____ (GOAL: TO FAILURE)   WEIGHT: _____
SET 4   REPS: _____ (GOAL: TO FAILURE)   WEIGHT: _____
(OPTIONAL)

SUPERSETS DONE TODAY (CIRCLE):
1   2   3   4

TODAY'S WORKOUT INTENSITY:
_____ / 10

EXERCISE
GUIDE
https://HabitNest.link/lifting24

Workout 24: Legs & Forearms

DATE _____

1. LEG PRESS
(ALTERNATIVE: DEADLIFT)

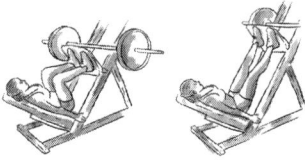

PREVIOUS BEST (WORKOUT 14)　REPS: _____　　　WEIGHT: _____

SET 1　REPS: _____ (GOAL: 10-15)　WEIGHT: _____
SET 2　REPS: _____ (GOAL: 8-12)　WEIGHT: _____
SET 3　REPS: _____ (GOAL: 6-8)　WEIGHT: _____
SET 4 (OPTIONAL)　REPS: _____ (GOAL: 4-6)　WEIGHT: _____

2. HACK SQUAT
(ALTERNATIVE: WEIGHTED LUNGE)

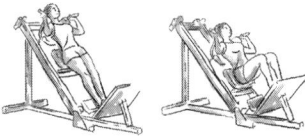

PREVIOUS BEST (WORKOUT 14)　REPS: _____　　　WEIGHT: _____

SET 1　REPS: _____ (GOAL: 10-15)　WEIGHT: _____
SET 2　REPS: _____ (GOAL: 8-12)　WEIGHT: _____
SET 3　REPS: _____ (GOAL: 6-8)　WEIGHT: _____
SET 4 (OPTIONAL)　REPS: _____ (GOAL: 4-6)　WEIGHT: _____

3. QUAD EXTENSION

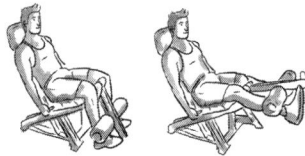

PREVIOUS BEST (WORKOUT 19)　REPS: _____　　　WEIGHT: _____

SET 1　REPS: _____ (GOAL: 10-15)　WEIGHT: _____
SET 2　REPS: _____ (GOAL: 8-12)　WEIGHT: _____
SET 3　REPS: _____ (GOAL: 6-8)　WEIGHT: _____
SET 4 (OPTIONAL)　REPS: _____ (GOAL: 4-6)　WEIGHT: _____

4. HAMSTRING EXTENSION

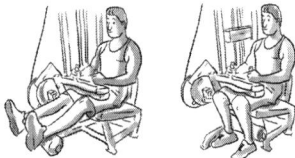

PREVIOUS BEST (WORKOUT 19)　REPS: _____　　　WEIGHT: _____

SET 1　REPS: _____ (GOAL: 10-15)　WEIGHT: _____
SET 2　REPS: _____ (GOAL: 8-12)　WEIGHT: _____
SET 3　REPS: _____ (GOAL: 6-8)　WEIGHT: _____
SET 4 (OPTIONAL)　REPS: _____ (GOAL: 4-6)　WEIGHT: _____

AMOUNT OF CARDIO DONE TODAY: _____

110

Workout 24: Legs & Forearms

5. CALF RAISE

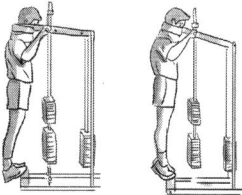

	PREVIOUS BEST (WORKOUT 19)	REPS: _____		WEIGHT: _____
SET 1		REPS: _____	(GOAL: 10-15)	WEIGHT: _____
SET 2		REPS: _____	(GOAL: 8-12)	WEIGHT: _____
SET 3		REPS: _____	(GOAL: 6-8)	WEIGHT: _____
SET 4 (OPTIONAL)		REPS: _____	(GOAL: 4-6)	WEIGHT: _____

1. REVERSE GRIP DUMBBELL CURL

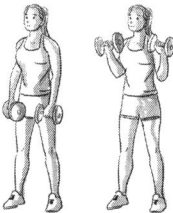

	PREVIOUS BEST (WORKOUT 19)	REPS: _____		WEIGHT: _____
SET 1		REPS: _____	(GOAL: 10-15)	WEIGHT: _____
SET 2		REPS: _____	(GOAL: 8-12)	WEIGHT: _____
SET 3		REPS: _____	(GOAL: 6-8)	WEIGHT: _____
SET 4 (OPTIONAL)		REPS: _____	(GOAL: 4-6)	WEIGHT: _____

2. DUMBBELL TWIST-UP

PREVIOUS BEST (WORKOUT 19)

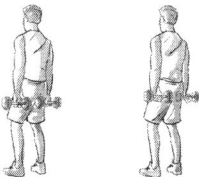

	REPS: _____		WEIGHT: _____
SET 1	REPS: _____	(GOAL: 10-15)	WEIGHT: _____
SET 2	REPS: _____	(GOAL: 8-12)	WEIGHT: _____
SET 3	REPS: _____	(GOAL: 6-8)	WEIGHT: _____
SET 4 (OPTIONAL)	REPS: _____	(GOAL: 4-6)	WEIGHT: _____

SUPERSETS DONE TODAY (CIRCLE):

1   2   3   4

TODAY'S WORKOUT INTENSITY:

_____ / 10

Workout 25: Full Body Circuit

DATE

Rest for **15-20 seconds** between each exercise, then rest for **1-2 minutes** after completing the entire circuit. Complete the full circuit **a total of 4-5 times.**

1. JUMPING JACK
(Duration: 30 Seconds)

2. AIR SQUAT
(Duration: 30 Seconds)

3. CRUNCH
(Duration: 30 Seconds)

4. MOUNTAIN CLIMBER
(Duration: 30 Seconds)

5. TOWEL PULL
(Duration: 30 Seconds)

6. HIGH KNEE
(Duration: 30 Seconds)

7. IN AND OUT PUSH-UP
(Duration: 30 Seconds)

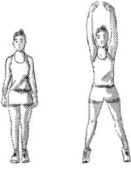

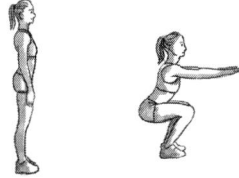

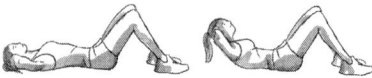

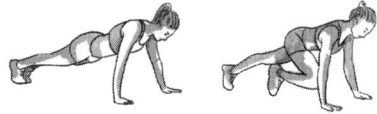

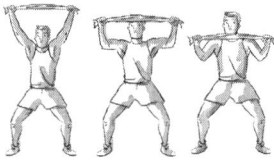

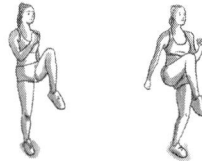

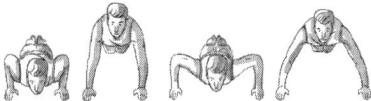

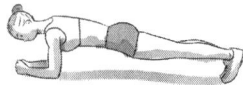

8. PLANK
(Duration: 30 Seconds)

<u>Double Pro-Tip</u> 💡

Experiment with increasing your protein intake.

Proper protein intake will make a significant, noticeable difference in your muscle growth. If you're not seeing as much muscle growth as you'd like, low protein intake could be the culprit.

As a reminder, a general standard amongst bodybuilders is to *intake 0.6-0.8 (or more) grams of protein per pound of body weight.* If you are overweight, you can instead intake 1gram per pound of lean body mass you have.

It's easy to dismiss this as being unreasonable or too hard to do, but with proper planning and food intake it becomes very doable. A large protein shake itself can provide up to 40g of protein. Adding this to your daily routine can help you hit your protein intake goals.

As always, first check with your doctor and/or a nutritionist to make sure you're okay in doing this. Intaking too much protein can lead to issues, as does having protein shakes with poor-quality ingredients.

If you are overweight, make getting lean your #1 priority.

When you are over a certain range of body fat (over 15% for males and 20% for females), your body is more likely to store excess calories as fat than as muscle.

If you fall above these ranges, you should make your first priority losing excess body fat (by being in a caloric deficit, doing consistent cardio, and doing resistance training).

Once you're leaner, you can pack on muscle much more efficiently.

Workout 26: Biceps & Shoulders

DATE _____

1. PREACHER CURL
(ALTERNATIVE: SEATED DUMBBELL CURL)

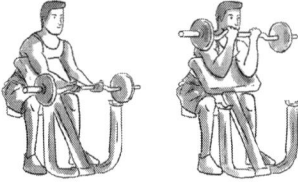

PREVIOUS BEST (WORKOUT 22) REPS: _____   WEIGHT: _____

SET 1	REPS: _____	(GOAL: 10-15)	WEIGHT: _____
SET 2	REPS: _____	(GOAL: 8-12)	WEIGHT: _____
SET 3	REPS: _____	(GOAL: 6-8)	WEIGHT: _____
SET 4 (OPTIONAL)	REPS: _____	(GOAL: 4-6)	WEIGHT: _____

2. ZOTTMAN CURL

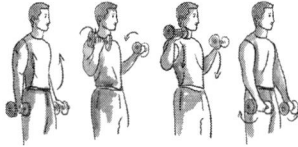

PREVIOUS BEST (WORKOUT 12) REPS: _____   WEIGHT: _____

SET 1	REPS: _____	(GOAL: 10-15)	WEIGHT: _____
SET 2	REPS: _____	(GOAL: 8-12)	WEIGHT: _____
SET 3	REPS: _____	(GOAL: 6-8)	WEIGHT: _____
SET 4 (OPTIONAL)	REPS: _____	(GOAL: 4-6)	WEIGHT: _____

3. UNDERHAND CABLE CURL

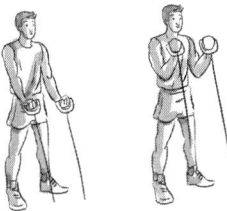

PREVIOUS BEST (WORKOUT 16) REPS: _____   WEIGHT: _____

SET 1	REPS: _____	(GOAL: 10-15)	WEIGHT: _____
SET 2	REPS: _____	(GOAL: 8-12)	WEIGHT: _____
SET 3	REPS: _____	(GOAL: 6-8)	WEIGHT: _____
SET 4 (OPTIONAL)	REPS: _____	(GOAL: 4-6)	WEIGHT: _____

4. ROPE HAMMER CURL

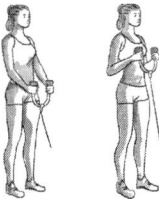

PREVIOUS BEST (WORKOUT 22) REPS: _____   WEIGHT: _____

SET 1	REPS: _____	(GOAL: 10-15)	WEIGHT: _____
SET 2	REPS: _____	(GOAL: 8-12)	WEIGHT: _____
SET 3	REPS: _____	(GOAL: 6-8)	WEIGHT: _____
SET 4 (OPTIONAL)	REPS: _____	(GOAL: 4-6)	WEIGHT: _____

AMOUNT OF CARDIO DONE TODAY: _____

Workout 26: Biceps & Shoulders

1. LATERAL DUMBBELL RAISE

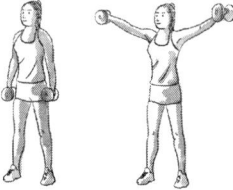

PREVIOUS BEST
(WORKOUT 23)   REPS: _____   WEIGHT: _____

SET 1   REPS: _____ (GOAL: 10-15)   WEIGHT: _____

SET 2   REPS: _____ (GOAL: 8-12)   WEIGHT: _____

SET 3   REPS: _____ (GOAL: 6-8)   WEIGHT: _____

SET 4   REPS: _____ (GOAL: 4-6)   WEIGHT: _____
(OPTIONAL)

2. FRONT DUMBBELL RAISE

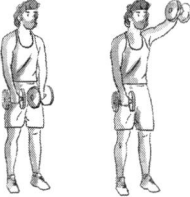

PREVIOUS BEST
(WORKOUT 13)   REPS: _____   WEIGHT: _____

SET 1   REPS: _____ (GOAL: 10-15)   WEIGHT: _____

SET 2   REPS: _____ (GOAL: 8-12)   WEIGHT: _____

SET 3   REPS: _____ (GOAL: 6-8)   WEIGHT: _____

SET 4   REPS: _____ (GOAL: 4-6)   WEIGHT: _____
(OPTIONAL)

3. BARBELL RAISE

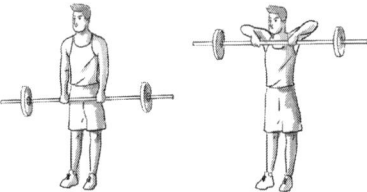

PREVIOUS BEST
(WORKOUT 23)   REPS: _____   WEIGHT: _____

SET 1   REPS: _____ (GOAL: 10-15)   WEIGHT: _____

SET 2   REPS: _____ (GOAL: 8-12)   WEIGHT: _____

SET 3   REPS: _____ (GOAL: 6-8)   WEIGHT: _____

SET 4   REPS: _____ (GOAL: 4-6)   WEIGHT: _____
(OPTIONAL)

4. ARNOLD DUMBBELL PRESS

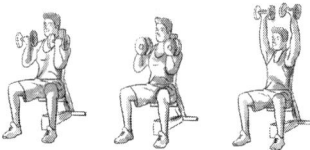

PREVIOUS BEST
(WORKOUT 18)   REPS: _____   WEIGHT: _____

SET 1   REPS: _____ (GOAL: 10-15)   WEIGHT: _____

SET 2   REPS: _____ (GOAL: 8-12)   WEIGHT: _____

SET 3   REPS: _____ (GOAL: 6-8)   WEIGHT: _____

SET 4   REPS: _____ (GOAL: 4-6)   WEIGHT: _____
(OPTIONAL)

SUPERSETS DONE TODAY (CIRCLE):

1   2   3   4

TODAY'S WORKOUT INTENSITY:

_____ / 10

Common Form Issue: **Back**

Problem

Your upper traps are tightened and bunched up.
This is a common way to ruin your back workout.

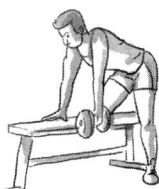

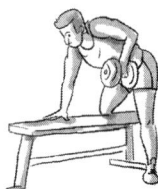

Improper Form

How to Fix This

Disengage your upper traps by lowering them as much as possible.
They should not be used at all. Your hands should hook on to the bar
and your back should do the pulling all by itself, no pulling with the
arms.

You may have to drastically lower the weight by ~50% if you have been
doing this improperly in the past. Your back should move the weight
forwards and backwards entirely, your arms should not be pulling the
weight at all.

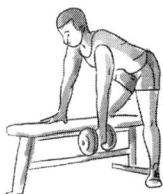

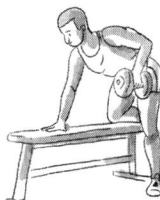

Proper Form

Exercises This Concept Applies To

All back exercises!

Common Form Issue: **Triceps**

(X)

Problem

Your elbows move at all during the movement.

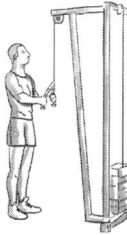

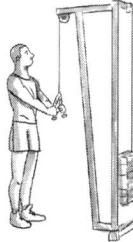

Improper Form

(✓)

How to Fix This

Keep your elbows completely stationary and allow your triceps to bear the entire load of the movement. If you can't do this, you're going too heavy and you're recruiting secondary muscles to help by moving your elbows.

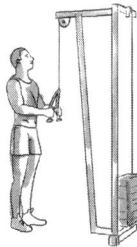

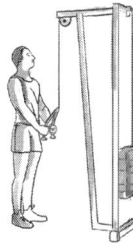

Proper Form

Exercises This Concept Applies To

Overhead Dumbbell Extension, Rope Pulldown, Skull Crusher, Close Grip Bench Press, Straight Bar Pulldown

Workout 27: Back & Triceps

DATE _____

1. ASSISTED PULL-UP

(ALTERNATIVE: PULL-UP OR TOWEL PULL)

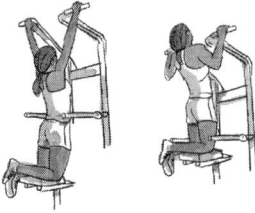

PREVIOUS BEST (WORKOUT 21)   REPS: _____   WEIGHT: _____

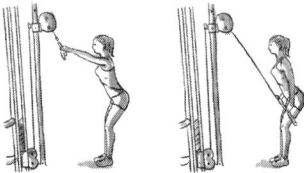

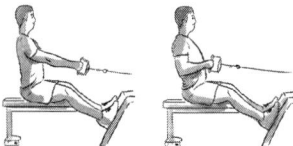

SET 1   REPS: _____   (GOAL: 10-15)   WEIGHT: _____

SET 2   REPS: _____   (GOAL: 8-12)   WEIGHT: _____

SET 3   REPS: _____   (GOAL: 6-8)   WEIGHT: _____

SET 4   REPS: _____   (GOAL: 4-6)   WEIGHT: _____
(OPTIONAL)

2. BENT OVER DUMBBELL ROW

PREVIOUS BEST (WORKOUT 21)   REPS: _____   WEIGHT: _____

(ALTERNATIVE: UPPER BACK ROPE PULL)

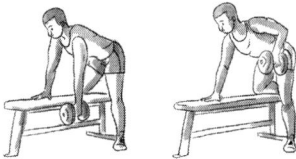

SET 1   REPS: _____   (GOAL: 10-15)   WEIGHT: _____

SET 2   REPS: _____   (GOAL: 8-12)   WEIGHT: _____

SET 3   REPS: _____   (GOAL: 6-8)   WEIGHT: _____

SET 4   REPS: _____   (GOAL: 4-6)   WEIGHT: _____
(OPTIONAL)

3. STRAIGHT ARM PULLDOWN

PREVIOUS BEST (WORKOUT 21)   REPS: _____   WEIGHT: _____

SET 1   REPS: _____   (GOAL: 10-15)   WEIGHT: _____

SET 2   REPS: _____   (GOAL: 8-12)   WEIGHT: _____

SET 3   REPS: _____   (GOAL: 6-8)   WEIGHT: _____

SET 4   REPS: _____   (GOAL: 4-6)   WEIGHT: _____
(OPTIONAL)

4. CLOSE GRIP CABLE ROW

(ALTERNATIVE: PULL-UP OR LAT ROW)

PREVIOUS BEST (WORKOUT 18)   REPS: _____   WEIGHT: _____

SET 1   REPS: _____   (GOAL: 10-15)   WEIGHT: _____

SET 2   REPS: _____   (GOAL: 8-12)   WEIGHT: _____

SET 3   REPS: _____   (GOAL: 6-8)   WEIGHT: _____

SET 4   REPS: _____   (GOAL: 4-6)   WEIGHT: _____
(OPTIONAL)

AMOUNT OF CARDIO DONE TODAY:
_____

Workout 27: Back & Triceps

1. SKULL CRUSHER
(ALTERNATIVE: DUMBBELL EXTENSION)

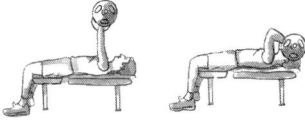

PREVIOUS BEST
(WORKOUT 23)

REPS: _____   WEIGHT: _____

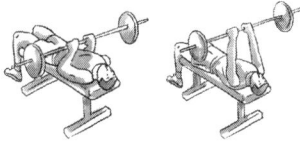

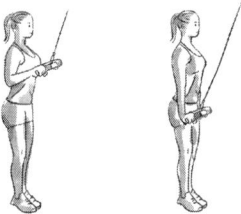

SET 1   REPS: _____ (GOAL: 10-15)   WEIGHT: _____
SET 2   REPS: _____ (GOAL: 8-12)   WEIGHT: _____
SET 3   REPS: _____ (GOAL: 6-8)   WEIGHT: _____
SET 4   REPS: _____ (GOAL: 4-6)   WEIGHT: _____
(OPTIONAL)

2. CLOSE GRIP BENCH PRESS
PREVIOUS BEST
(WORKOUT 13)

REPS: _____   WEIGHT: _____

SET 1   REPS: _____ (GOAL: 10-15)   WEIGHT: _____
SET 2   REPS: _____ (GOAL: 8-12)   WEIGHT: _____
SET 3   REPS: _____ (GOAL: 6-8)   WEIGHT: _____
SET 4   REPS: _____ (GOAL: 4-6)   WEIGHT: _____
(OPTIONAL)

3. STRAIGHT BAR PULLDOWN
PREVIOUS BEST
(WORKOUT 6)

REPS: _____   WEIGHT: _____

SET 1   REPS: _____ (GOAL: 10-15)   WEIGHT: _____
SET 2   REPS: _____ (GOAL: 8-12)   WEIGHT: _____
SET 3   REPS: _____ (GOAL: 6-8)   WEIGHT: _____
SET 4   REPS: _____ (GOAL: 4-6)   WEIGHT: _____
(OPTIONAL)

4. DIAMOND PUSH-UP
(ALTERNATIVE: ASSISTED DIP
OR SEATED DIP W/ MACHINE)

PREVIOUS BEST
(WORKOUT 13)

REPS: _____

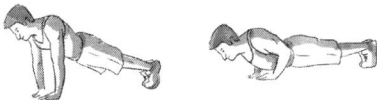

SET 1   REPS: _____ (GOAL: TO FAILURE)
SET 2   REPS: _____ (GOAL: TO FAILURE)
SET 3   REPS: _____ (GOAL: TO FAILURE)
SET 4   REPS: _____ (GOAL: TO FAILURE)
(OPTIONAL)

SUPERSETS DONE TODAY (CIRCLE):
1   2   3   4

TODAY'S WORKOUT INTENSITY:
_____ / 10

119

Workout 28: Chest & Forearms

DATE _____

1. FLAT BENCH PRESS

(ALTERNATIVE: FLAT BENCH DUMBBELL PRESS)

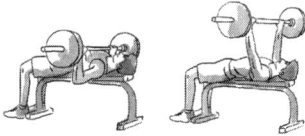

PREVIOUS BEST
(WORKOUT 22)   REPS: _____   WEIGHT: _____

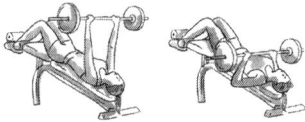

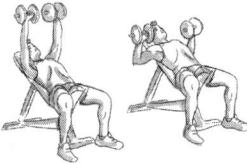

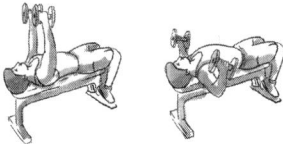

SET 1	REPS: _____	(GOAL: 10-15)	WEIGHT: _____
SET 2	REPS: _____	(GOAL: 8-12)	WEIGHT: _____
SET 3	REPS: _____	(GOAL: 6-8)	WEIGHT: _____
SET 4 (OPTIONAL)	REPS: _____	(GOAL: 4-6)	WEIGHT: _____

2. DECLINE BENCH PRESS

PREVIOUS BEST
(WORKOUT 17)   REPS: _____   WEIGHT: _____

SET 1	REPS: _____	(GOAL: 10-15)	WEIGHT: _____
SET 2	REPS: _____	(GOAL: 8-12)	WEIGHT: _____
SET 3	REPS: _____	(GOAL: 6-8)	WEIGHT: _____
SET 4 (OPTIONAL)	REPS: _____	(GOAL: 4-6)	WEIGHT: _____

3. INCLINE DUMBBELL PRESS

(ALTERNATIVE: INCLINE BENCH PRESS)

PREVIOUS BEST
(WORKOUT 12)   REPS: _____   WEIGHT: _____

SET 1	REPS: _____	(GOAL: 10-15)	WEIGHT: _____
SET 2	REPS: _____	(GOAL: 8-12)	WEIGHT: _____
SET 3	REPS: _____	(GOAL: 6-8)	WEIGHT: _____
SET 4 (OPTIONAL)	REPS: _____	(GOAL: 4-6)	WEIGHT: _____

4. FLAT BENCH DUMBBELL FLY

(ALTERNATIVE: CHEST FLY W/ MACHINE)

PREVIOUS BEST
(WORKOUT 12)   REPS: _____   WEIGHT: _____

SET 1	REPS: _____	(GOAL: 10-15)	WEIGHT: _____
SET 2	REPS: _____	(GOAL: 8-12)	WEIGHT: _____
SET 3	REPS: _____	(GOAL: 6-8)	WEIGHT: _____
SET 4 (OPTIONAL)	REPS: _____	(GOAL: 4-6)	WEIGHT: _____

AMOUNT OF CARDIO DONE TODAY: _____

Workout 28: Chest & Forearms

5. CABLE CROSSOVER
(ALTERNATIVE: FLAT BENCH DUMBBELL PRESS)

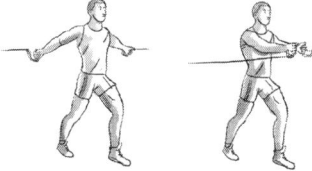

PREVIOUS BEST [WORKOUT 17]

REPS: _____   WEIGHT: _____

SET 1	REPS: _____	(GOAL: 10-15)	WEIGHT: _____
SET 2	REPS: _____	(GOAL: 8-12)	WEIGHT: _____
SET 3	REPS: _____	(GOAL: 6-8)	WEIGHT: _____
SET 4 [OPTIONAL]	REPS: _____	(GOAL: 4-6)	WEIGHT: _____

1. REVERSE GRIP EZ BAR CURL
(ALTERNATIVE: FARMER'S WALK)

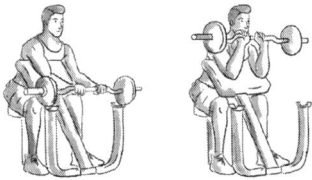

PREVIOUS BEST [WORKOUT 8]

REPS: _____   WEIGHT: _____

SET 1	REPS: _____	(GOAL: 10-15)	WEIGHT: _____
SET 2	REPS: _____	(GOAL: 8-12)	WEIGHT: _____
SET 3	REPS: _____	(GOAL: 6-8)	WEIGHT: _____
SET 4 [OPTIONAL]	REPS: _____	(GOAL: 4-6)	WEIGHT: _____

2. BARBELL TWIST-UP
(ALTERNATIVE: PULL-UP BAR HANG)

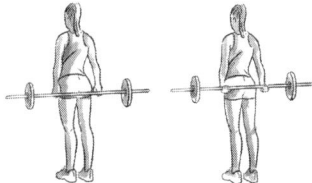

PREVIOUS BEST [WORKOUT 8]

REPS: _____   WEIGHT: _____

SET 1	REPS: _____	(GOAL: 10-15)	WEIGHT: _____
SET 2	REPS: _____	(GOAL: 8-12)	WEIGHT: _____
SET 3	REPS: _____	(GOAL: 6-8)	WEIGHT: _____
SET 4 [OPTIONAL]	REPS: _____	(GOAL: 4-6)	WEIGHT: _____

TODAY'S WORKOUT INTENSITY:
_____ / 10

EXERCISE
GUIDE
https://HabitNest.link/lifting29

Workout 29: Legs & Abs

DATE _____

1. DEADLIFT
(ALTERNATIVE: LEG PRESS)

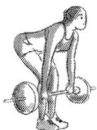

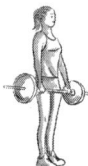

	PREVIOUS BEST (WORKOUT 19)	REPS: _____		WEIGHT: _____
	SET 1	REPS: _____	(GOAL: 10-15)	WEIGHT: _____
	SET 2	REPS: _____	(GOAL: 8-12)	WEIGHT: _____
	SET 3	REPS: _____	(GOAL: 6-8)	WEIGHT: _____
	SET 4 (OPTIONAL)	REPS: _____	(GOAL: 4-6)	WEIGHT: _____

2. BARBELL SQUAT
(ALTERNATIVE: HACK SQUAT)

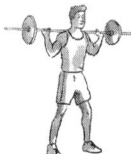

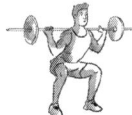

	PREVIOUS BEST (WORKOUT 19)	REPS: _____		WEIGHT: _____
	SET 1	REPS: _____	(GOAL: 10-15)	WEIGHT: _____
	SET 2	REPS: _____	(GOAL: 8-12)	WEIGHT: _____
	SET 3	REPS: _____	(GOAL: 6-8)	WEIGHT: _____
	SET 4 (OPTIONAL)	REPS: _____	(GOAL: 4-6)	WEIGHT: _____

3. WEIGHTED LUNGE
(ALTERNATIVE: QUAD EXTENSION)

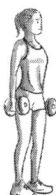

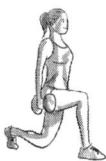

	PREVIOUS BEST (WORKOUT 14)	REPS: _____		WEIGHT: _____
	SET 1	REPS: _____	(GOAL: 10-15)	WEIGHT: _____
	SET 2	REPS: _____	(GOAL: 8-12)	WEIGHT: _____
	SET 3	REPS: _____	(GOAL: 6-8)	WEIGHT: _____
	SET 4 (OPTIONAL)	REPS: _____	(GOAL: 4-6)	WEIGHT: _____

4. HAMSTRING EXTENSION

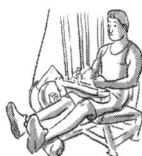

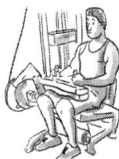

	PREVIOUS BEST (WORKOUT 24)	REPS: _____		WEIGHT: _____
	SET 1	REPS: _____	(GOAL: 10-15)	WEIGHT: _____
	SET 2	REPS: _____	(GOAL: 8-12)	WEIGHT: _____
	SET 3	REPS: _____	(GOAL: 6-8)	WEIGHT: _____
	SET 4 (OPTIONAL)	REPS: _____	(GOAL: 4-6)	WEIGHT: _____

AMOUNT OF CARDIO DONE TODAY: _____

122

<u>Workout 29: Legs & Abs</u>

5. CALF RAISE

(ALTERNATIVE: SEATED CALF PRESS MACHINE)

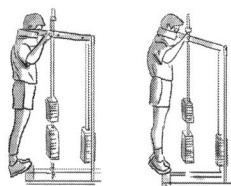

PREVIOUS BEST (WORKOUT 24)	REPS: _____		WEIGHT: _____
SET 1	REPS: _____	(GOAL: 10-15)	WEIGHT: _____
SET 2	REPS: _____	(GOAL: 8-12)	WEIGHT: _____
SET 3	REPS: _____	(GOAL: 6-8)	WEIGHT: _____
SET 4 (OPTIONAL)	REPS: _____	(GOAL: 4-6)	WEIGHT: _____

1. KNEELING CABLE CRUNCH

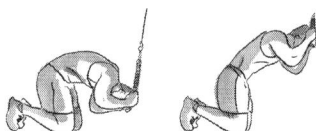

PREVIOUS BEST (WORKOUT 21)	REPS: _____		WEIGHT: _____
SET 1	REPS: _____	(GOAL: 10-20)	WEIGHT: _____
SET 2	REPS: _____	(GOAL: 10-20)	WEIGHT: _____
SET 3	REPS: _____	(GOAL: 10-20)	WEIGHT: _____

2. HANGING LEG LIFT

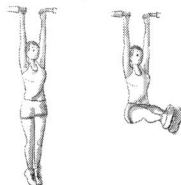

PREVIOUS BEST (WORKOUT 14)	REPS: _____	
SET 1	REPS: _____	(GOAL: 10-20)
SET 2	REPS: _____	(GOAL: 10-20)
SET 3	REPS: _____	(GOAL: 10-20)

3. STARFISH CRUNCH

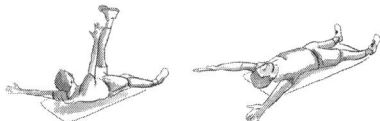

PREVIOUS BEST (WORKOUT 21)	REPS: _____	
SET 1	REPS: _____	(GOAL: 10-20 EACH SIDE)
SET 2	REPS: _____	(GOAL: 10-20 EACH SIDE)
SET 3	REPS: _____	(GOAL: 10-20 EACH SIDE)

4. PLANK

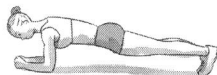

PREVIOUS BEST (WORKOUT 17)	TIME: _____	
SET 1	TIME: _____	(GOAL: 45-90 SECONDS)
SET 2	TIME: _____	(GOAL: 45-90 SECONDS)
SET 3	TIME: _____	(GOAL: 45-90 SECONDS)

SUPERSETS DONE TODAY (CIRCLE):

1   2   3   4

TODAY'S WORKOUT INTENSITY:

_____ / 10

Workout 30: Full Body Circuit

*Rest for **15-20 seconds** between each exercise, then rest for **1-2 minutes** after completing the entire circuit. Complete the full circuit **a total of 4-5 times.***

1. RUN IN PLACE

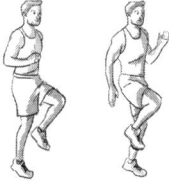

(Duration: 30 Seconds)

2. ALTERNATING LUNGE

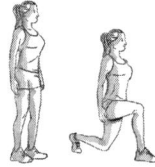

(Duration: 30 Seconds)

3. STARFISH CRUNCH

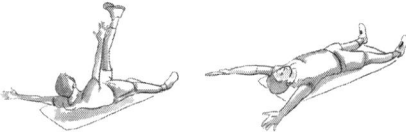

(Duration: 30 Seconds)

4. TOWEL SNATCH

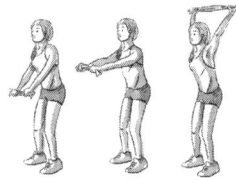

(Duration: 30 Seconds)

5. PUSH-UP

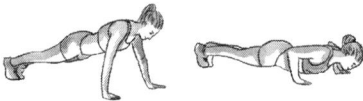

(Duration: 30 Seconds)

6. HIGH KNEE

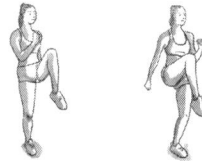

(Duration: 30 Seconds)

7. BURPEE

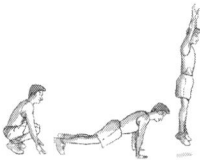

(Duration: 30 Seconds)

8. BICYCLE CRUNCH

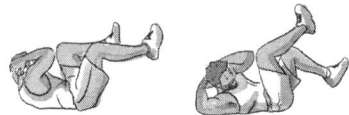

(Duration: 30 Seconds)

Check-In

How do I feel about the way I look now compared to when I started?

_____

_____

_____

_____

Which body parts am I happier with?

_____

_____

_____

_____

Which body parts do I need to work more (maybe a bonus day for those muscles)?

_____

_____

_____

_____

Am I noticing any changes in my mental attitude in general (happier, more confident, etc.)?

_____

_____

_____

_____

Bonus Challenge

Going forward, complete all four sets of four exercises instead of three.

So far in the book, we left the number of sets for each exercise as three, with the fourth being listed as optional.

This is because looking at so many sets may be overwhelming for many (8 exercises with 4 sets each = 32 sets a day!)

And it is. It's undeniably a lot of volume to pack into a workout.

But performing enough volume during workouts is one of the major keys to hypertrophy. So challenge yourself to complete four sets of four of the exercises that show up each day.

If you feel overwhelmed by this thought, consider that some of the best bodybuilders in the world perform **two full workouts a day** (yes, even those not using performance enhancing drugs).

Although that extent of exercise is a bit extreme, the results serve as a testament to the effectiveness of additional workout volume.

(Optional)
I will complete all four sets of four exercises for the next week.

_____   _____
Signature   Date

Workout 31: Chest & Abs

DATE _____

1. FLAT BENCH PRESS
(ALTERNATIVE: FLAT BENCH DUMBBELL PRESS)

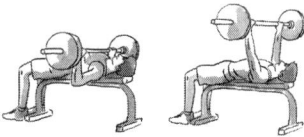

PREVIOUS BEST
(WORKOUT 28)

REPS: _____   WEIGHT: _____

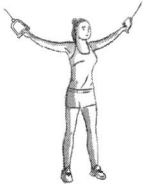

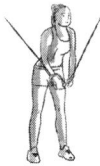

SET 1	REPS: _____	(GOAL: 10-15)	WEIGHT: _____
SET 2	REPS: _____	(GOAL: 8-12)	WEIGHT: _____
SET 3	REPS: _____	(GOAL: 6-8)	WEIGHT: _____
SET 4 (OPTIONAL)	REPS: _____	(GOAL: 4-6)	WEIGHT: _____

2. HIGH TO LOW CABLE FLY

PREVIOUS BEST
(WORKOUT 22)

REPS: _____   WEIGHT: _____

SET 1	REPS: _____	(GOAL: 10-15)	WEIGHT: _____
SET 2	REPS: _____	(GOAL: 8-12)	WEIGHT: _____
SET 3	REPS: _____	(GOAL: 6-8)	WEIGHT: _____
SET 4 (OPTIONAL)	REPS: _____	(GOAL: 4-6)	WEIGHT: _____

3. INCLINE DUMBBELL PRESS
(ALTERNATIVE: INCLINE BENCH PRESS)

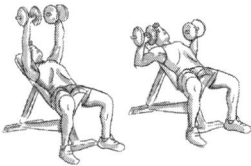

PREVIOUS BEST
(WORKOUT 28)

REPS: _____   WEIGHT: _____

SET 1	REPS: _____	(GOAL: 10-15)	WEIGHT: _____
SET 2	REPS: _____	(GOAL: 8-12)	WEIGHT: _____
SET 3	REPS: _____	(GOAL: 6-8)	WEIGHT: _____
SET 4 (OPTIONAL)	REPS: _____	(GOAL: 4-6)	WEIGHT: _____

4. FLAT BENCH DUMBBELL FLY
(ALTERNATIVE: CHEST FLY W/ MACHINE)

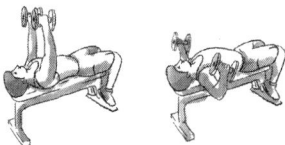

PREVIOUS BEST
(WORKOUT 28)

REPS: _____   WEIGHT: _____

SET 1	REPS: _____	(GOAL: 10-15)	WEIGHT: _____
SET 2	REPS: _____	(GOAL: 8-12)	WEIGHT: _____
SET 3	REPS: _____	(GOAL: 6-8)	WEIGHT: _____
SET 4 (OPTIONAL)	REPS: _____	(GOAL: 4-6)	WEIGHT: _____

AMOUNT OF CARDIO DONE TODAY: _____

Workout 31: Chest & Abs

5. LOW TO HIGH CABLE FLY

(ALTERNATIVE: SEATED CALF PRESS MACHINE)

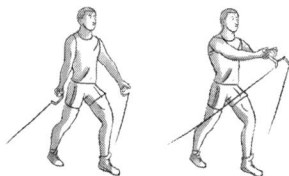

PREVIOUS BEST
(WORKOUT 22)

SET 1 REPS: _____ (GOAL: 10-15)   WEIGHT: _____

SET 2 REPS: _____ (GOAL: 8-12)   WEIGHT: _____

SET 3 REPS: _____ (GOAL: 6-8)   WEIGHT: _____

SET 4 REPS: _____ (GOAL: 4-6)   WEIGHT: _____
(OPTIONAL)

1. KNEELING CABLE CRUNCH

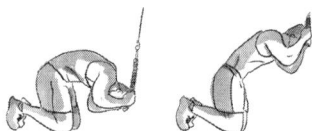

PREVIOUS BEST REPS: _____   WEIGHT: _____
(WORKOUT 29)

SET 1 REPS: _____ (GOAL: 10-20)   WEIGHT: _____

SET 2 REPS: _____ (GOAL: 10-20)   WEIGHT: _____

SET 3 REPS: _____ (GOAL: 10-20)   WEIGHT: _____

2. BICYCLE CRUNCH

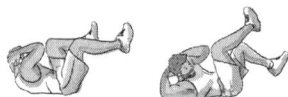

PREVIOUS BEST REPS: _____
(WORKOUT 21)

SET 1 REPS: _____ (GOAL: 10-20 EACH SIDE)

SET 2 REPS: _____ (GOAL: 10-20 EACH SIDE)

SET 3 REPS: _____ (GOAL: 10-20 EACH SIDE)

3. RUSSIAN TWIST

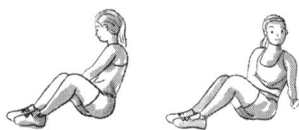

PREVIOUS BEST REPS: _____
(WORKOUT 21)

SET 1 REPS: _____ (GOAL: 10-20 EACH SIDE)

SET 2 REPS: _____ (GOAL: 10-20 EACH SIDE)

SET 3 REPS: _____ (GOAL: 10-20 EACH SIDE)

4. PLANK

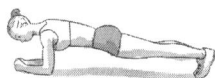

PREVIOUS BEST TIME: _____
(WORKOUT 29)

SET 1 TIME: _____ (GOAL: 45-90 SECONDS)

SET 2 TIME: _____ (GOAL: 45-90 SECONDS)

SET 3 TIME: _____ (GOAL: 45-90 SECONDS)

SUPERSETS DONE TODAY (CIRCLE):
1   2   3   4

TODAY'S WORKOUT INTENSITY:
_____ / 10

Workout 32: Back & Biceps

1. ASSISTED PULL-UP
(ALTERNATIVE: PULL-UP OR TOWEL PULL)

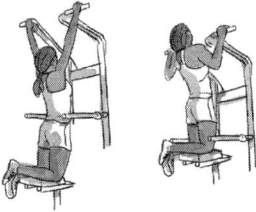

PREVIOUS BEST
(WORKOUT 27)

REPS: _____   WEIGHT: _____

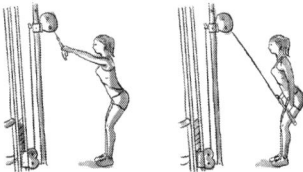

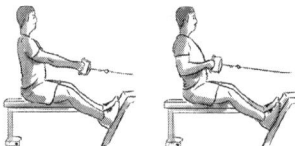

SET 1	REPS: _____	(GOAL: 10-15)	WEIGHT: _____
SET 2	REPS: _____	(GOAL: 8-12)	WEIGHT: _____
SET 3	REPS: _____	(GOAL: 6-8)	WEIGHT: _____
SET 4 (OPTIONAL)	REPS: _____	(GOAL: 4-6)	WEIGHT: _____

2. T-BAR ROW
(ALTERNATIVE: UPPER BACK ROPE PULL)

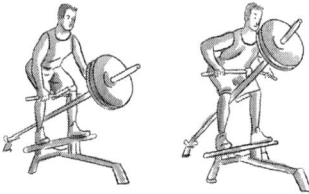

PREVIOUS BEST
(WORKOUT 18)

REPS: _____   WEIGHT: _____

SET 1	REPS: _____	(GOAL: 10-15)	WEIGHT: _____
SET 2	REPS: _____	(GOAL: 8-12)	WEIGHT: _____
SET 3	REPS: _____	(GOAL: 6-8)	WEIGHT: _____
SET 4 (OPTIONAL)	REPS: _____	(GOAL: 4-6)	WEIGHT: _____

3. STRAIGHT ARM PULLDOWN

PREVIOUS BEST
(WORKOUT 27)

REPS: _____   WEIGHT: _____

SET 1	REPS: _____	(GOAL: 10-15)	WEIGHT: _____
SET 2	REPS: _____	(GOAL: 8-12)	WEIGHT: _____
SET 3	REPS: _____	(GOAL: 6-8)	WEIGHT: _____
SET 4 (OPTIONAL)	REPS: _____	(GOAL: 4-6)	WEIGHT: _____

4. CLOSE GRIP CABLE ROW
(ALTERNATIVE: PULL-UP OR LAT ROW)

PREVIOUS BEST
(WORKOUT 27)

REPS: _____   WEIGHT: _____

SET 1	REPS: _____	(GOAL: 10-15)	WEIGHT: _____
SET 2	REPS: _____	(GOAL: 8-12)	WEIGHT: _____
SET 3	REPS: _____	(GOAL: 6-8)	WEIGHT: _____
SET 4 (OPTIONAL)	REPS: _____	(GOAL: 4-6)	WEIGHT: _____

AMOUNT OF CARDIO DONE TODAY:

Workout 32: Back & Biceps

1. PREACHER CURL
(ALTERNATIVE: SEATED DUMBBELL CURL)

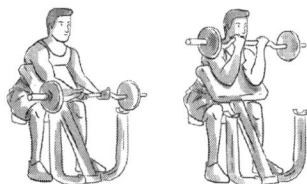

PREVIOUS BEST (WORKOUT 26)
REPS: _____   WEIGHT: _____

SET 1 REPS: _____ (GOAL: 10-15)   WEIGHT: _____
SET 2 REPS: _____ (GOAL: 8-12)   WEIGHT: _____
SET 3 REPS: _____ (GOAL: 6-8)   WEIGHT: _____
SET 4 REPS: _____ (GOAL: 4-6)   WEIGHT: _____
(OPTIONAL)

2. ZOTTMAN CURL

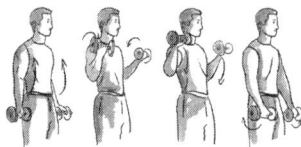

PREVIOUS BEST (WORKOUT 26)
REPS: _____   WEIGHT: _____

SET 1 REPS: _____ (GOAL: 10-15)   WEIGHT: _____
SET 2 REPS: _____ (GOAL: 8-12)   WEIGHT: _____
SET 3 REPS: _____ (GOAL: 6-8)   WEIGHT: _____
SET 4 REPS: _____ (GOAL: 4-6)   WEIGHT: _____
(OPTIONAL)

3. ROPE HAMMER CURL

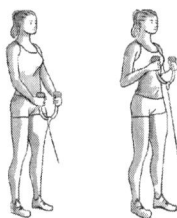

PREVIOUS BEST (WORKOUT 26)
REPS: _____   WEIGHT: _____

SET 1 REPS: _____ (GOAL: 10-15)   WEIGHT: _____
SET 2 REPS: _____ (GOAL: 8-12)   WEIGHT: _____
SET 3 REPS: _____ (GOAL: 6-8)   WEIGHT: _____
SET 4 REPS: _____ (GOAL: 4-6)   WEIGHT: _____
(OPTIONAL)

4. UNDERHAND CABLE CURL

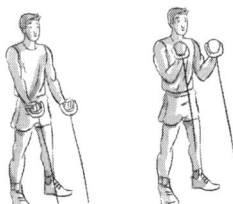

PREVIOUS BEST (WORKOUT 26)
REPS: _____   WEIGHT: _____

SET 1 REPS: _____ (GOAL: 10-15)   WEIGHT: _____
SET 2 REPS: _____ (GOAL: 8-12)   WEIGHT: _____
SET 3 REPS: _____ (GOAL: 6-8)   WEIGHT: _____
SET 4 REPS: _____ (GOAL: 4-6)   WEIGHT: _____
(OPTIONAL)

SUPERSETS DONE TODAY (CIRCLE):
1   2   3   4

TODAY'S WORKOUT INTENSITY:
_____ / 10

Common Form Issue: **Shoulders**

Problem

You're swinging your shoulders and using your lifting momentum throughout the movement.

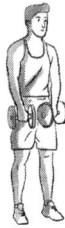

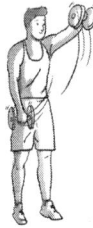

Improper Form

How to Fix This

Try performing the entirety of the movement (all the way up, all the way down) with full control on the weight and without swinging your arms.

If you can't hit the recommended rep ranges, consider lowering the weight.

Note: Focus on your mind-muscle connection to CONTROL the movement at every second of each lift, both upwards and downwards.

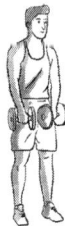

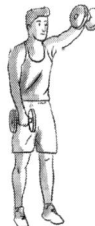

Proper Form

Exercises This Concept Applies To

All Shoulder Exercises (Except Shrugs)!

Common Form Issue: **Triceps**

Problem

(X)

Your lats are not engaged / tightened to keep them in place and allow your tricep to bear the load of your movement.

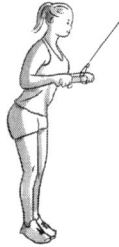

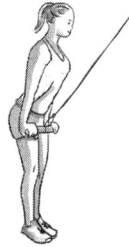

Improper Form

How to Fix This

(✓)

Pull your upper back together, keep your lats engaged, keep your elbow in place, and only allow your triceps to move the weight.

Note: If you have weak rear delts or lats, you may feel it particularly in those muscles instead of your triceps until they catch up strength wise.

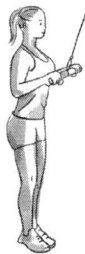

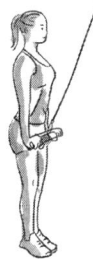

Proper Form

Exercises This Concept Applies To

Rope Pulldown, Skull Crusher, Dip

Workout 33: Shoulders & Triceps

DATE _____

1. BARBELL RAISE

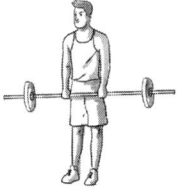

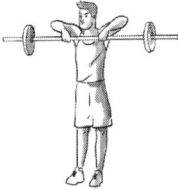

PREVIOUS BEST
(WORKOUT 26)   REPS: _____   WEIGHT: _____

SET 1   REPS: _____ (GOAL: 10-15)   WEIGHT: _____

SET 2   REPS: _____ (GOAL: 8-12)   WEIGHT: _____

SET 3   REPS: _____ (GOAL: 6-8)   WEIGHT: _____

SET 4
(OPTIONAL)   REPS: _____ (GOAL: 4-6)   WEIGHT: _____

2. FRONT DUMBBELL RAISE

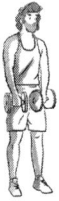

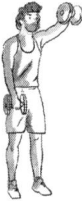

PREVIOUS BEST
(WORKOUT 26)   REPS: _____   WEIGHT: _____

SET 1   REPS: _____ (GOAL: 10-15)   WEIGHT: _____

SET 2   REPS: _____ (GOAL: 8-12)   WEIGHT: _____

SET 3   REPS: _____ (GOAL: 6-8)   WEIGHT: _____

SET 4
(OPTIONAL)   REPS: _____ (GOAL: 4-6)   WEIGHT: _____

3. REVERSE FLY

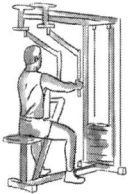

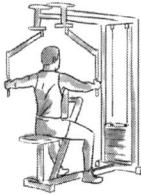

PREVIOUS BEST
(WORKOUT 23)   REPS: _____   WEIGHT: _____

SET 1   REPS: _____ (GOAL: 10-15)   WEIGHT: _____

SET 2   REPS: _____ (GOAL: 8-12)   WEIGHT: _____

SET 3   REPS: _____ (GOAL: 6-8)   WEIGHT: _____

SET 4
(OPTIONAL)   REPS: _____ (GOAL: 4-6)   WEIGHT: _____

4. SEATED DUMBBELL PRESS

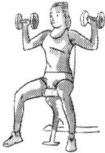

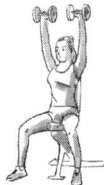

PREVIOUS BEST
(WORKOUT 23)   REPS: _____   WEIGHT: _____

SET 1   REPS: _____ (GOAL: 10-15)   WEIGHT: _____

SET 2   REPS: _____ (GOAL: 8-12)   WEIGHT: _____

SET 3   REPS: _____ (GOAL: 6-8)   WEIGHT: _____

SET 4
(OPTIONAL)   REPS: _____ (GOAL: 4-6)   WEIGHT: _____

AMOUNT OF CARDIO DONE TODAY: _____

Workout 33: Shoulders & Triceps

1. SKULL CRUSHER

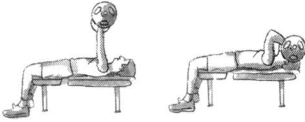

PREVIOUS BEST (WORKOUT 27)	REPS: _____		WEIGHT: _____
SET 1	REPS: _____	(GOAL: 10-15)	WEIGHT: _____
SET 2	REPS: _____	(GOAL: 8-12)	WEIGHT: _____
SET 3	REPS: _____	(GOAL: 6-8)	WEIGHT: _____
SET 4 (OPTIONAL)	REPS: _____	(GOAL: 4-6)	WEIGHT: _____

2. CLOSE GRIP BENCH PRESS

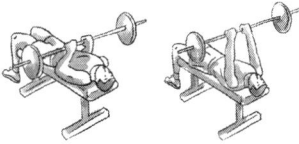

PREVIOUS BEST (WORKOUT 27)	REPS: _____		WEIGHT: _____
SET 1	REPS: _____	(GOAL: 10-15)	WEIGHT: _____
SET 2	REPS: _____	(GOAL: 8-12)	WEIGHT: _____
SET 3	REPS: _____	(GOAL: 6-8)	WEIGHT: _____
SET 4 (OPTIONAL)	REPS: _____	(GOAL: 4-6)	WEIGHT: _____

3. ROPE PULLDOWN

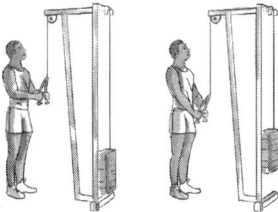

PREVIOUS BEST (WORKOUT 23)	REPS: _____		WEIGHT: _____
SET 1	REPS: _____	(GOAL: 10-15)	WEIGHT: _____
SET 2	REPS: _____	(GOAL: 8-12)	WEIGHT: _____
SET 3	REPS: _____	(GOAL: 6-8)	WEIGHT: _____
SET 4 (OPTIONAL)	REPS: _____	(GOAL: 4-6)	WEIGHT: _____

4. DIP

(ALTERNATIVE: ASSISTED DIP OR SEATED DIP W/ MACHINE)

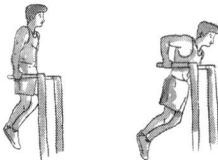

PREVIOUS BEST (WORKOUT 23)	REPS: _____		WEIGHT: _____
SET 1	REPS: _____	(GOAL: TO FAILURE)	WEIGHT: _____
SET 2	REPS: _____	(GOAL: TO FAILURE)	WEIGHT: _____
SET 3	REPS: _____	(GOAL: TO FAILURE)	WEIGHT: _____
SET 4 (OPTIONAL)	REPS: _____	(GOAL: TO FAILURE)	WEIGHT: _____

SUPERSETS DONE TODAY (CIRCLE):

1   2   3   4

TODAY'S WORKOUT INTENSITY:

_____ / 10

Workout 34: Legs & Abs

1. LEG PRESS
(ALTERNATIVE: DEADLIFT)

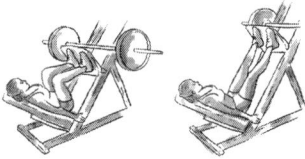

PREVIOUS BEST (WORKOUT 24) REPS: _____   WEIGHT: _____

SET 1   REPS: _____ (GOAL: 10-15)   WEIGHT: _____
SET 2   REPS: _____ (GOAL: 8-12)   WEIGHT: _____
SET 3   REPS: _____ (GOAL: 6-8)   WEIGHT: _____
SET 4 (OPTIONAL)   REPS: _____ (GOAL: 4-6)   WEIGHT: _____

2. HACK SQUAT
(ALTERNATIVE: WEIGHTED LUNGE)

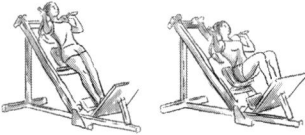

PREVIOUS BEST (WORKOUT 24) REPS: _____   WEIGHT: _____

SET 1   REPS: _____ (GOAL: 10-15)   WEIGHT: _____
SET 2   REPS: _____ (GOAL: 8-12)   WEIGHT: _____
SET 3   REPS: _____ (GOAL: 6-8)   WEIGHT: _____
SET 4 (OPTIONAL)   REPS: _____ (GOAL: 4-6)   WEIGHT: _____

3. QUAD EXTENSION

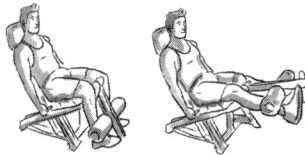

PREVIOUS BEST (WORKOUT 24) REPS: _____   WEIGHT: _____

SET 1   REPS: _____ (GOAL: 10-15)   WEIGHT: _____
SET 2   REPS: _____ (GOAL: 8-12)   WEIGHT: _____
SET 3   REPS: _____ (GOAL: 6-8)   WEIGHT: _____
SET 4 (OPTIONAL)   REPS: _____ (GOAL: 4-6)   WEIGHT: _____

4. HAMSTRING EXTENSION

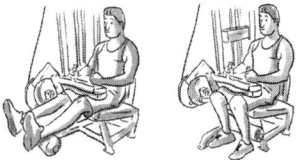

PREVIOUS BEST (WORKOUT 29) REPS: _____   WEIGHT: _____

SET 1   REPS: _____ (GOAL: 10-15)   WEIGHT: _____
SET 2   REPS: _____ (GOAL: 8-12)   WEIGHT: _____
SET 3   REPS: _____ (GOAL: 6-8)   WEIGHT: _____
SET 4 (OPTIONAL)   REPS: _____ (GOAL: 4-6)   WEIGHT: _____

AMOUNT OF CARDIO DONE TODAY: _____

Workout 34: Legs & Abs

5. CALF RAISE

(ALTERNATIVE: SEATED CALF PRESS MACHINE)

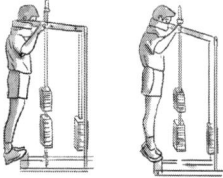

PREVIOUS BEST (WORKOUT 29) REPS: _____ WEIGHT: _____

SET 1 REPS: _____ (GOAL: 10-15) WEIGHT: _____

SET 2 REPS: _____ (GOAL: 8-12) WEIGHT: _____

SET 3 REPS: _____ (GOAL: 6-8) WEIGHT: _____

SET 4 (OPTIONAL) REPS: _____ (GOAL: 4-6) WEIGHT: _____

1. KNEELING CABLE CRUNCH

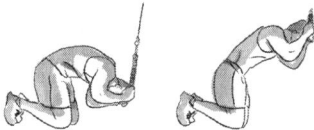

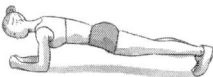

PREVIOUS BEST (WORKOUT 31) REPS: _____ WEIGHT: _____

SET 1 REPS: _____ (GOAL: 10-20) WEIGHT: _____

SET 2 REPS: _____ (GOAL: 10-20) WEIGHT: _____

SET 3 REPS: _____ (GOAL: 10-20) WEIGHT: _____

2. LEG LIFT

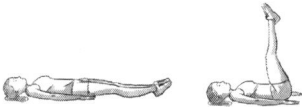

PREVIOUS BEST (WORKOUT 17) REPS: _____

SET 1 REPS: _____ (GOAL: 10-20)

SET 2 REPS: _____ (GOAL: 10-20)

SET 3 REPS: _____ (GOAL: 10-20)

3. STARFISH CRUNCH

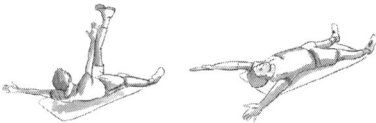

PREVIOUS BEST (WORKOUT 29) REPS: _____

SET 1 REPS: _____ (GOAL: 10-20 EACH SIDE)

SET 2 REPS: _____ (GOAL: 10-20 EACH SIDE)

SET 3 REPS: _____ (GOAL: 10-20 EACH SIDE)

4. PLANK

PREVIOUS BEST (WORKOUT 31) TIME: _____

SET 1 TIME: _____ (GOAL: 45-90 SECONDS)

SET 2 TIME: _____ (GOAL: 45-90 SECONDS)

SET 3 TIME: _____ (GOAL: 45-90 SECONDS)

SUPERSETS DONE TODAY (CIRCLE):

1   2   3   4

137

TODAY'S WORKOUT INTENSITY:

_____ / 10

Workout 35: Full Body Circuit

DATE _____

Rest for 15-20 seconds between each exercise, then rest for 1-2 minutes after completing the entire circuit. Complete the full circuit a total of 4-5 times.

1. JUMP

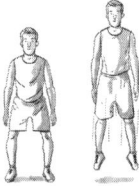

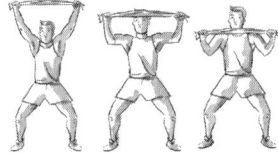

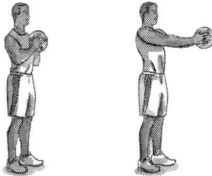

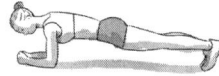

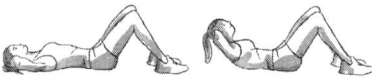

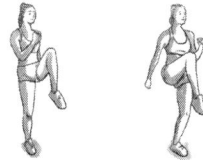

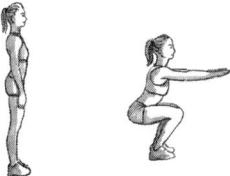

(Duration: 30 Seconds)

2. TOWEL PULL

(Duration: 30 Seconds)

3. PRAYER

(Duration: 30 Seconds)

4. PLANK

(Duration: 30 Seconds)

5. CRUNCH

(Duration: 30 Seconds)

6. HIGH KNEE

(Duration: 30 Seconds)

7. AIR SQUAT

(Duration: 30 Seconds)

8. VERTICAL LEAP

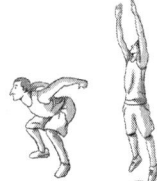

(Duration: 30 Seconds)

TODAY'S WORKOUT INTENSITY:

_____ / 10

Super Read

> *Read "Burn The Fat, Feed The Muscle" by Tom Venuto*

Disclaimer: We have no affiliation with Tom Venuto or his book and aren't getting paid in any way for this recommendation. It's simply a great tool.

Certain points of this journal were influenced by his book, and for good reason.

Burn The Fat, Feed The Muscle is one of the most thorough, scientifically-based books out there on fitness and nutrition.

Venuto gives all the best information out there that has been battle tested with hundreds of people and boiled down to only the most effective tips.

To take it a step further, he always creates clear, easy-to-follow action steps for most problems you'll face along this journey. He covers these for lifters of all stages - beginner, intermediate, or advanced.

If you feel it would be useful for you to have a very thorough breakdown of all this, you can find his book on Amazon. It comes as a printed hardcopy, Kindle version for your phone/tablet, or audiobook.

Workout 36: Shoulders & Biceps

1. LATERAL DUMBBELL RAISE

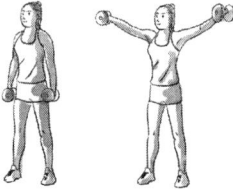

PREVIOUS BEST (WORKOUT 26)	REPS: _____	WEIGHT: _____
SET 1	REPS: _____ (GOAL: 10-15)	WEIGHT: _____
SET 2	REPS: _____ (GOAL: 8-12)	WEIGHT: _____
SET 3	REPS: _____ (GOAL: 6-8)	WEIGHT: _____
SET 4 (OPTIONAL)	REPS: _____ (GOAL: 4-6)	WEIGHT: _____

2. ARNOLD DUMBBELL PRESS

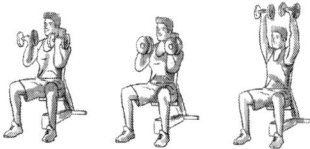

PREVIOUS BEST (WORKOUT 26)	REPS: _____	WEIGHT: _____
SET 1	REPS: _____ (GOAL: 10-15)	WEIGHT: _____
SET 2	REPS: _____ (GOAL: 8-12)	WEIGHT: _____
SET 3	REPS: _____ (GOAL: 6-8)	WEIGHT: _____
SET 4 (OPTIONAL)	REPS: _____ (GOAL: 4-6)	WEIGHT: _____

3. REVERSE FLY

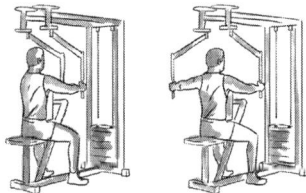

PREVIOUS BEST (WORKOUT 33)	REPS: _____	WEIGHT: _____
SET 1	REPS: _____ (GOAL: 10-15)	WEIGHT: _____
SET 2	REPS: _____ (GOAL: 8-12)	WEIGHT: _____
SET 3	REPS: _____ (GOAL: 6-8)	WEIGHT: _____
SET 4 (OPTIONAL)	REPS: _____ (GOAL: 4-6)	WEIGHT: _____

4. BARBELL RAISE

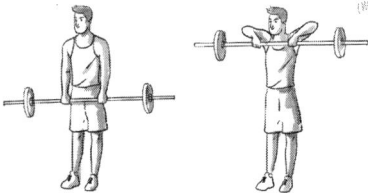

PREVIOUS BEST (WORKOUT 33)	REPS: _____	WEIGHT: _____
SET 1	REPS: _____ (GOAL: 10-15)	WEIGHT: _____
SET 2	REPS: _____ (GOAL: 8-12)	WEIGHT: _____
SET 3	REPS: _____ (GOAL: 6-8)	WEIGHT: _____
SET 4 (OPTIONAL)	REPS: _____ (GOAL: 4-6)	WEIGHT: _____

AMOUNT OF CARDIO DONE TODAY:

Workout 36: Shoulders & Biceps

1. PREACHER CURL

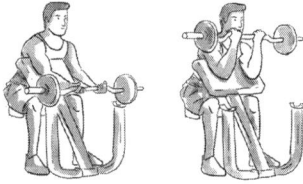

PREVIOUS BEST (WORKOUT 32)	REPS: _____		WEIGHT: _____
SET 1	REPS: _____	(GOAL: 10-15)	WEIGHT: _____
SET 2	REPS: _____	(GOAL: 8-12)	WEIGHT: _____
SET 3	REPS: _____	(GOAL: 6-8)	WEIGHT: _____
SET 4 (OPTIONAL)	REPS: _____	(GOAL: 4-6)	WEIGHT: _____

2. ZOTTMAN CURL

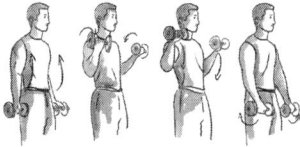

PREVIOUS BEST (WORKOUT 32)	REPS: _____		WEIGHT: _____
SET 1	REPS: _____	(GOAL: 10-15)	WEIGHT: _____
SET 2	REPS: _____	(GOAL: 8-12)	WEIGHT: _____
SET 3	REPS: _____	(GOAL: 6-8)	WEIGHT: _____
SET 4 (OPTIONAL)	REPS: _____	(GOAL: 4-6)	WEIGHT: _____

3. CONCENTRATION CURL

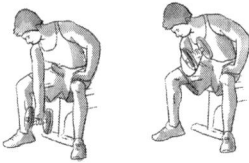

PREVIOUS BEST (WORKOUT 16)	REPS: _____		WEIGHT: _____
SET 1	REPS: _____	(GOAL: 10-15)	WEIGHT: _____
SET 2	REPS: _____	(GOAL: 8-12)	WEIGHT: _____
SET 3	REPS: _____	(GOAL: 6-8)	WEIGHT: _____
SET 4 (OPTIONAL)	REPS: _____	(GOAL: 4-6)	WEIGHT: _____

4. OVERHEAD CABLE CURL

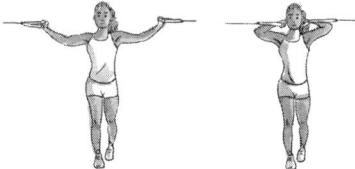

PREVIOUS BEST (WORKOUT 22)	REPS: _____		WEIGHT: _____
SET 1	REPS: _____	(GOAL: 10-15)	WEIGHT: _____
SET 2	REPS: _____	(GOAL: 8-12)	WEIGHT: _____
SET 3	REPS: _____	(GOAL: 6-8)	WEIGHT: _____
SET 4 (OPTIONAL)	REPS: _____	(GOAL: 4-6)	WEIGHT: _____

SUPERSETS DONE TODAY (CIRCLE):

1   2   3   4

TODAY'S WORKOUT INTENSITY:

_____ / 10

Workout 37: Chest & Abs

DATE _____

1. FLAT BENCH PRESS

(ALTERNATIVE: FLAT BENCH DUMBBELL PRESS)

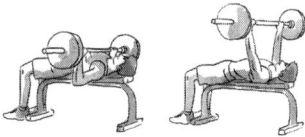

PREVIOUS BEST (WORKOUT 31)   REPS: _____   WEIGHT: _____

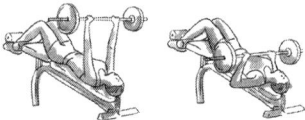

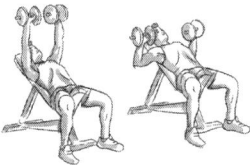

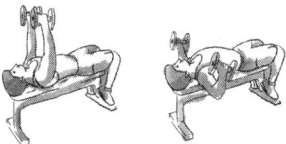

SET 1	REPS: _____ (GOAL: 10-15)	WEIGHT: _____
SET 2	REPS: _____ (GOAL: 8-12)	WEIGHT: _____
SET 3	REPS: _____ (GOAL: 6-8)	WEIGHT: _____
SET 4 (OPTIONAL)		

2. DECLINE BENCH PRESS

PREVIOUS BEST (WORKOUT 28)   REPS: _____   WEIGHT: _____

SET 1	REPS: _____ (GOAL: 10-15)	WEIGHT: _____
SET 2	REPS: _____ (GOAL: 8-12)	WEIGHT: _____
SET 3	REPS: _____ (GOAL: 6-8)	WEIGHT: _____
SET 4 (OPTIONAL)	REPS: _____ (GOAL: 4-6)	WEIGHT: _____

3. INCLINE DUMBBELL PRESS

(ALTERNATIVE: INCLINE BENCH PRESS)

PREVIOUS BEST (WORKOUT 31)   REPS: _____   WEIGHT: _____

SET 1	REPS: _____ (GOAL: 10-15)	WEIGHT: _____
SET 2	REPS: _____ (GOAL: 8-12)	WEIGHT: _____
SET 3	REPS: _____ (GOAL: 6-8)	WEIGHT: _____
SET 4 (OPTIONAL)	REPS: _____ (GOAL: 4-6)	WEIGHT: _____

4. FLAT BENCH DUMBBELL FLY

PREVIOUS BEST (WORKOUT 31)   REPS: _____   WEIGHT: _____

SET 1	REPS: _____ (GOAL: 10-15)	WEIGHT: _____
SET 2	REPS: _____ (GOAL: 8-12)	WEIGHT: _____
SET 3	REPS: _____ (GOAL: 6-8)	WEIGHT: _____
SET 4 (OPTIONAL)	REPS: _____ (GOAL: 4-6)	WEIGHT: _____

AMOUNT OF CARDIO DONE TODAY: _____

Workout 37: Chest & Abs

5. CABLE CROSSOVER

(ALTERNATIVE: CHEST FLY W/ MACHINE)

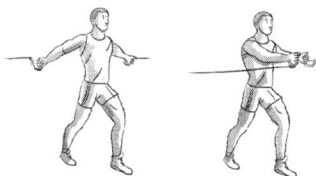

PREVIOUS BEST (WORKOUT 28)	REPS: _____		WEIGHT: _____
SET 1	REPS: _____	(GOAL: 10-15)	WEIGHT: _____
SET 2	REPS: _____	(GOAL: 8-12)	WEIGHT: _____
SET 3	REPS: _____	(GOAL: 6-8)	WEIGHT: _____
SET 4 (OPTIONAL)	REPS: _____	(GOAL: 4-6)	WEIGHT: _____

1. KNEELING CABLE CRUNCH

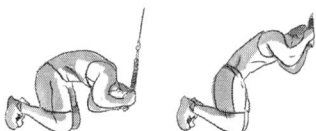

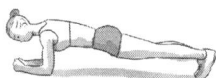

PREVIOUS BEST (WORKOUT 34)	REPS: _____		WEIGHT: _____
SET 1	REPS: _____	(GOAL: 10-20)	WEIGHT: _____
SET 2	REPS: _____	(GOAL: 10-20)	WEIGHT: _____
SET 3	REPS: _____	(GOAL: 10-20)	WEIGHT: _____

2. HANGING LEG LIFT

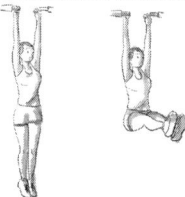

PREVIOUS BEST (WORKOUT 29)	REPS: _____	
SET 1	REPS: _____	(GOAL: 10-20)
SET 2	REPS: _____	(GOAL: 10-20)
SET 3	REPS: _____	(GOAL: 10-20)

3. BICYCLE CRUNCH

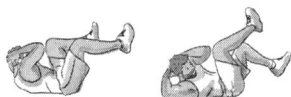

PREVIOUS BEST (WORKOUT 31)	REPS: _____	
SET 1	REPS: _____	(GOAL: 10-20 EACH SIDE)
SET 2	REPS: _____	(GOAL: 10-20 EACH SIDE)
SET 3	REPS: _____	(GOAL: 10-20 EACH SIDE)

4. PLANK

PREVIOUS BEST (WORKOUT 34)	TIME: _____	
SET 1	TIME: _____	(GOAL: 45-90 SECONDS)
SET 2	TIME: _____	(GOAL: 45-90 SECONDS)
SET 3	TIME: _____	(GOAL: 45-90 SECONDS)

SUPERSETS DONE TODAY (CIRCLE):

1   2   3   4

143

TODAY'S WORKOUT INTENSITY:

_____ / 10

EXERCISE
GUIDE
https://HabitNest.link/lifting38

Workout 38: Back & Triceps

DATE _____

1. ASSISTED PULL-UP
(ALTERNATIVE: PULL-UP OR TOWEL PULL)

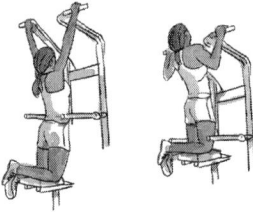

PREVIOUS BEST (WORKOUT 32)   REPS: _____   WEIGHT: _____

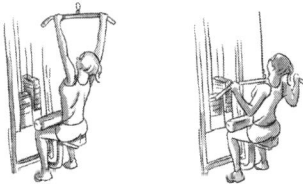

SET 1   REPS: _____ (GOAL: 10-15)   WEIGHT: _____
SET 2   REPS: _____ (GOAL: 8-12)   WEIGHT: _____
SET 3   REPS: _____ (GOAL: 6-8)   WEIGHT: _____
SET 4   REPS: _____ (GOAL: 4-6)   WEIGHT: _____
(OPTIONAL)

2. T-BAR ROW
(ALTERNATIVE: UPPER BACK ROPE PULL)

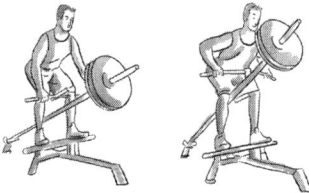

PREVIOUS BEST (WORKOUT 32)   REPS: _____   WEIGHT: _____

SET 1   REPS: _____ (GOAL: 10-15)   WEIGHT: _____
SET 2   REPS: _____ (GOAL: 8-12)   WEIGHT: _____
SET 3   REPS: _____ (GOAL: 6-8)   WEIGHT: _____
SET 4   REPS: _____ (GOAL: 4-6)   WEIGHT: _____
(OPTIONAL)

3. LAT PULLDOWN

PREVIOUS BEST (WORKOUT 18)   REPS: _____   WEIGHT: _____

SET 1   REPS: _____ (GOAL: 10-15)   WEIGHT: _____
SET 2   REPS: _____ (GOAL: 8-12)   WEIGHT: _____
SET 3   REPS: _____ (GOAL: 6-8)   WEIGHT: _____
SET 4   REPS: _____ (GOAL: 4-6)   WEIGHT: _____
(OPTIONAL)

4. CLOSE GRIP CABLE ROW
(ALTERNATIVE: PULL-UP OR LAT ROW)

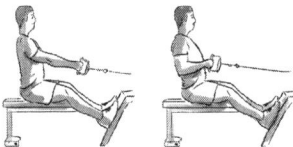

PREVIOUS BEST (WORKOUT 32)   REPS: _____   WEIGHT: _____

SET 1   REPS: _____ (GOAL: 10-15)   WEIGHT: _____
SET 2   REPS: _____ (GOAL: 8-12)   WEIGHT: _____
SET 3   REPS: _____ (GOAL: 6-8)   WEIGHT: _____
SET 4   REPS: _____ (GOAL: 4-6)   WEIGHT: _____
(OPTIONAL)

AMOUNT OF CARDIO DONE TODAY: _____

144

<u>Workout 38:</u> Back & **Triceps**

1. CLOSE GRIP BENCH PRESS
(ALTERNATIVE: DUMBBELL PULLOVER)

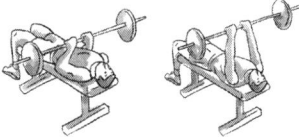

PREVIOUS BEST
(WORKOUT 33)   REPS: _____   WEIGHT: _____

SET 1   REPS: _____   (GOAL: 10-15)   WEIGHT: _____

SET 2   REPS: _____   (GOAL: 8-12)   WEIGHT: _____

SET 3   REPS: _____   (GOAL: 6-8)   WEIGHT: _____

SET 4   REPS: _____   (GOAL: 4-6)   WEIGHT: _____
(OPTIONAL)

(You can do this exercise seated if that's more comfortable for you.)

2. OVERHEAD DUMBBELL EXTENSION

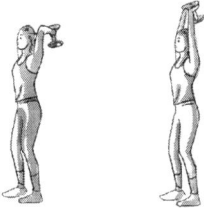

PREVIOUS BEST
(WORKOUT 23)   REPS: _____   WEIGHT: _____

SET 1   REPS: _____   (GOAL: 10-15)   WEIGHT: _____

SET 2   REPS: _____   (GOAL: 8-12)   WEIGHT: _____

SET 3   REPS: _____   (GOAL: 6-8)   WEIGHT: _____

SET 4   REPS: _____   (GOAL: 4-6)   WEIGHT: _____
(OPTIONAL)

3. ROPE PULLDOWN

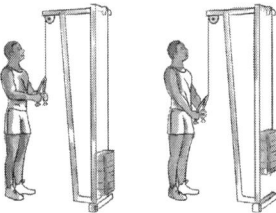

PREVIOUS BEST
(WORKOUT 33)   REPS: _____   WEIGHT: _____

SET 1   REPS: _____   (GOAL: 10-15)   WEIGHT: _____

SET 2   REPS: _____   (GOAL: 8-12)   WEIGHT: _____

SET 3   REPS: _____   (GOAL: 6-8)   WEIGHT: _____

SET 4   REPS: _____   (GOAL: 4-6)   WEIGHT: _____
(OPTIONAL)

4. DIP
(ALTERNATIVE: ASSISTED DIP
OR SEATED DIP W/ MACHINE)

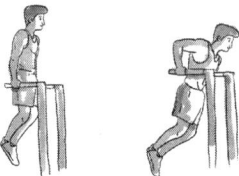

PREVIOUS BEST
(WORKOUT 33)   REPS: _____   WEIGHT: _____

SET 1   REPS: _____   (GOAL: TO FAILURE)   WEIGHT: _____

SET 2   REPS: _____   (GOAL: TO FAILURE)   WEIGHT: _____

SET 3   REPS: _____   (GOAL: TO FAILURE)   WEIGHT: _____

SET 4   REPS: _____   (GOAL: TO FAILURE)   WEIGHT: _____
(OPTIONAL)

SUPERSETS DONE TODAY (CIRCLE):
1   2   3   4

TODAY'S WORKOUT INTENSITY:
_____ / 10

Workout 39: Legs & Abs

DATE _____

1. DEADLIFT

(ALTERNATIVE: LEG PRESS)

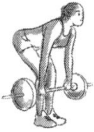

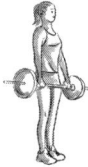

PREVIOUS BEST (WORKOUT 29)	REPS: _____	WEIGHT: _____
SET 1	REPS: _____ (GOAL: 10-15)	WEIGHT: _____
SET 2	REPS: _____ (GOAL: 8-12)	WEIGHT: _____
SET 3	REPS: _____ (GOAL: 6-8)	WEIGHT: _____
SET 4 (OPTIONAL)	REPS: _____ (GOAL: 4-6)	WEIGHT: _____

2. BARBELL SQUAT

(ALTERNATIVE: HACK SQUAT)

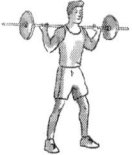

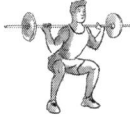

PREVIOUS BEST (WORKOUT 29)	REPS: _____	WEIGHT: _____
SET 1	REPS: _____ (GOAL: 10-15)	WEIGHT: _____
SET 2	REPS: _____ (GOAL: 8-12)	WEIGHT: _____
SET 3	REPS: _____ (GOAL: 6-8)	WEIGHT: _____
SET 4 (OPTIONAL)	REPS: _____ (GOAL: 4-6)	WEIGHT: _____

3. QUAD EXTENSION

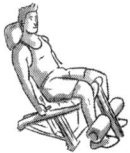

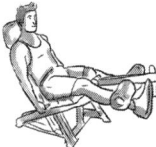

PREVIOUS BEST (WORKOUT 34)	REPS: _____	WEIGHT: _____
SET 1	REPS: _____ (GOAL: 10-15)	WEIGHT: _____
SET 2	REPS: _____ (GOAL: 8-12)	WEIGHT: _____
SET 3	REPS: _____ (GOAL: 6-8)	WEIGHT: _____
SET 4 (OPTIONAL)	REPS: _____ (GOAL: 4-6)	WEIGHT: _____

4. HAMSTRING EXTENSION

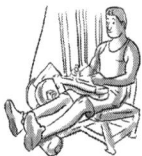

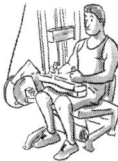

PREVIOUS BEST (WORKOUT 34)	REPS: _____	WEIGHT: _____
SET 1	REPS: _____ (GOAL: 10-15)	WEIGHT: _____
SET 2	REPS: _____ (GOAL: 8-12)	WEIGHT: _____
SET 3	REPS: _____ (GOAL: 6-8)	WEIGHT: _____
SET 4 (OPTIONAL)	REPS: _____ (GOAL: 4-6)	WEIGHT: _____

AMOUNT OF CARDIO DONE TODAY:

_____

Workout 39: Legs & Abs

5. CALF RAISE

(ALTERNATIVE: SEATED CALF PRESS MACHINE)

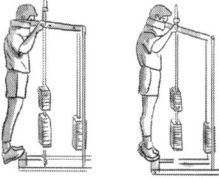

PREVIOUS BEST (WORKOUT 34)	REPS: _____		WEIGHT: _____
SET 1	REPS: _____	(GOAL: 10-15)	WEIGHT: _____
SET 2	REPS: _____	(GOAL: 8-12)	WEIGHT: _____
SET 3	REPS: _____	(GOAL: 6-8)	WEIGHT: _____
SET 4 (OPTIONAL)	REPS: _____	(GOAL: 4-6)	WEIGHT: _____

1. KNEELING CABLE CRUNCH

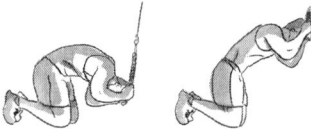

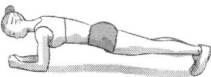

PREVIOUS BEST (WORKOUT 37)	REPS: _____		WEIGHT: _____
SET 1	REPS: _____	(GOAL: 10-20)	WEIGHT: _____
SET 2	REPS: _____	(GOAL: 10-20)	WEIGHT: _____
SET 3	REPS: _____	(GOAL: 10-20)	WEIGHT: _____

2. HANGING LEG LIFT

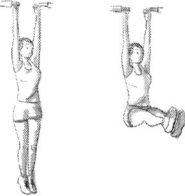

PREVIOUS BEST (WORKOUT 37)	REPS: _____	
SET 1	REPS: _____	(GOAL: 10-20)
SET 2	REPS: _____	(GOAL: 10-20)
SET 3	REPS: _____	(GOAL: 10-20)

3. STARFISH CRUNCH

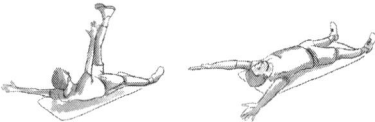

PREVIOUS BEST (WORKOUT 34)	REPS: _____	
SET 1	REPS: _____	(GOAL: 10-20 EACH SIDE)
SET 2	REPS: _____	(GOAL: 10-20 EACH SIDE)
SET 3	REPS: _____	(GOAL: 10-20 EACH SIDE)

4. PLANK

PREVIOUS BEST (WORKOUT 37)	TIME: _____	
SET 1	TIME: _____	(GOAL: 45-90 SECONDS)
SET 2	TIME: _____	(GOAL: 45-90 SECONDS)
SET 3	TIME: _____	(GOAL: 45-90 SECONDS)

SUPERSETS DONE TODAY (CIRCLE):

1   2   3   4

TODAY'S WORKOUT INTENSITY:

_____ / 10

Workout 40: Full Body Circuit

Rest for **15-20 seconds** between each exercise, then rest for **1-2 minutes** after completing the entire circuit. Complete the full circuit **a total of 4-5 times.**

1. JUMPING JACK
(Duration: 30 Seconds)

2. MOUNTAIN CLIMBER
(Duration: 30 Seconds)

3. STARFISH CRUNCH
(Duration: 30 Seconds)

4. SIDE PLANK
(Duration: 30 Seconds)

5. ALTERNATING LUNGE
(Duration: 30 Seconds)

6. TOWEL SNATCH
(Duration: 30 Seconds)

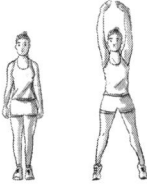

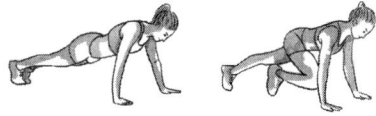

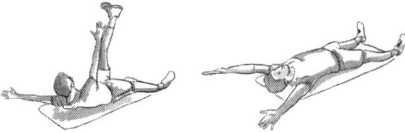

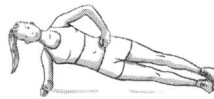

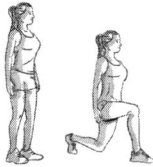

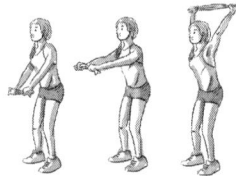

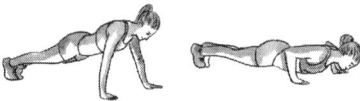

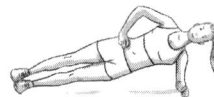

7. PUSH-UP
(Duration: 30 Seconds)

8. SIDE PLANK
(Duration: 30 Seconds)

TODAY'S WORKOUT INTENSITY:
_____ / 10

<u>Check-In</u>

When I'm in the middle of an exercise, am I mentally connected with the muscles that are being worked? How can I increase the quality of my mind-muscle connection during exercises?

_____

_____

_____

_____

Am I spending enough time focusing on the body parts I'm least satisfied with?

_____

_____

_____

_____

What do I love most about working out consistently?

_____

_____

_____

_____

How has my view of myself changed now that I've completed 40 workouts?

_____

_____

_____

_____

Bonus Challenge

> *Set a long-term goal to master your eating choices one step at a time.*

You already know that being on top of your nutrition goals will make a significant difference on how your body takes shape. But having perfect nutrition goes way past your body's physical manifestation.

Your daily nutrients are the source of your body's energy. The upside of mastering your nutrition is insane.

Although we built our *Nutrition Sidekick Journal* as a guide for this journey of mastery, it's not a necessity to make major shifts in your eating.

If you are not eating perfectly, there is always a reason - usually multiple. Instead of trying to change all of these eating habits at once (which is incredibly hard and impractical), we invite you to approach the process by **mastering one long-lasting change at a time.**

You may have dozens of little eating habits to change. To list some out:

- *A desire to finish everything on your plate*
- *A feeling that 'food is special / rare' and not to waste rare opportunities to eat specially-prepared food*
- *A feeling that because you ate so well during the week that you deserve to indulge more over the weekend*
- *That if your body is signaling a mood to eat something, the right move is to follow that impulse*

These are all untrue paradigms. Once you realize how to break each of them, your eyes will open to *how much happier* you can be. You will have an utter mastery of food choices and your energy.

You'll be able to walk into ANY situation, any event, and not be ruled by food, which ultimately serves YOU and your body. OWN your food, own your food choices, and you will slowly build your undeniable power over it.

Food mastery is a life-changing skill that will affect you for the rest of your life and serve as your rocket to the land of incredible physique, confidence, health, vitality, and energy.

With one change at a time you will begin to see the momentum, impact, and level of ultimate control you have over your body and your future. Use this fuel to help feed your growth and decision making.

(Optional)
I will commit to being mindful of every food choice I make this week.

Signature	Date

Workout 41: Biceps & Triceps

DATE _____

1. PREACHER CURL
(ALTERNATIVE: SEATED DUMBBELL CURL)

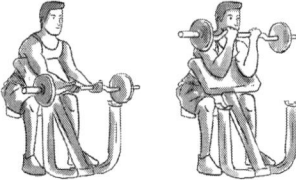

PREVIOUS BEST
(WORKOUT 36)

REPS: _____   WEIGHT: _____

SET 1	REPS: _____	(GOAL: 10-15)	WEIGHT: _____
SET 2	REPS: _____	(GOAL: 8-12)	WEIGHT: _____
SET 3	REPS: _____	(GOAL: 6-8)	WEIGHT: _____
SET 4 (OPTIONAL)	REPS: _____	(GOAL: 4-6)	WEIGHT: _____

2. ZOTTMAN CURL

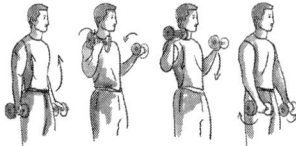

PREVIOUS BEST
(WORKOUT 36)

REPS: _____   WEIGHT: _____

SET 1	REPS: _____	(GOAL: 10-15)	WEIGHT: _____
SET 2	REPS: _____	(GOAL: 8-12)	WEIGHT: _____
SET 3	REPS: _____	(GOAL: 6-8)	WEIGHT: _____
SET 4 (OPTIONAL)	REPS: _____	(GOAL: 4-6)	WEIGHT: _____

3. UNDERHAND CABLE CURL

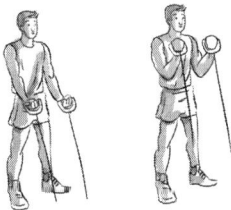

PREVIOUS BEST
(WORKOUT 32)

REPS: _____   WEIGHT: _____

SET 1	REPS: _____	(GOAL: 10-15)	WEIGHT: _____
SET 2	REPS: _____	(GOAL: 8-12)	WEIGHT: _____
SET 3	REPS: _____	(GOAL: 6-8)	WEIGHT: _____
SET 4 (OPTIONAL)	REPS: _____	(GOAL: 4-6)	WEIGHT: _____

4. ROPE HAMMER CURL

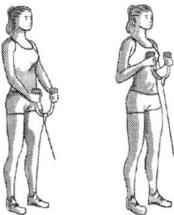

PREVIOUS BEST
(WORKOUT 32)

REPS: _____   WEIGHT: _____

SET 1	REPS: _____	(GOAL: 10-15)	WEIGHT: _____
SET 2	REPS: _____	(GOAL: 8-12)	WEIGHT: _____
SET 3	REPS: _____	(GOAL: 6-8)	WEIGHT: _____
SET 4 (OPTIONAL)	REPS: _____	(GOAL: 4-6)	WEIGHT: _____

AMOUNT OF CARDIO DONE TODAY: _____

Workout 41: Biceps & Triceps

1. SKULL CRUSHER
(ALTERNATIVE: CLOSE GRIP BENCH PRESS OR DUMBBELL PULLOVER)

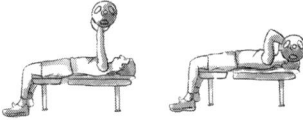

PREVIOUS BEST (WORKOUT 33)   REPS: _____   WEIGHT: _____

SET 1   REPS: _____   (GOAL: 10-15)   WEIGHT: _____
SET 2   REPS: _____   (GOAL: 8-12)   WEIGHT: _____
SET 3   REPS: _____   (GOAL: 6-8)   WEIGHT: _____
SET 4 (OPTIONAL)   REPS: _____   (GOAL: 4-6)   WEIGHT: _____

2. OVERHEAD DUMBBELL EXTENSION

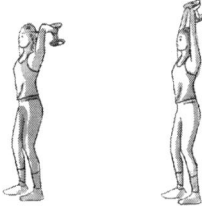

PREVIOUS BEST (WORKOUT 38)   REPS: _____   WEIGHT: _____

SET 1   REPS: _____   (GOAL: 10-15)   WEIGHT: _____
SET 2   REPS: _____   (GOAL: 8-12)   WEIGHT: _____
SET 3   REPS: _____   (GOAL: 6-8)   WEIGHT: _____
SET 4 (OPTIONAL)   REPS: _____   (GOAL: 4-6)   WEIGHT: _____

3. ROPE PULLDOWN

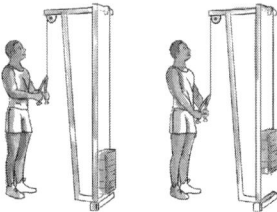

PREVIOUS BEST (WORKOUT 38)   REPS: _____   WEIGHT: _____

SET 1   REPS: _____   (GOAL: 10-15)   WEIGHT: _____
SET 2   REPS: _____   (GOAL: 8-12)   WEIGHT: _____
SET 3   REPS: _____   (GOAL: 6-8)   WEIGHT: _____
SET 4 (OPTIONAL)   REPS: _____   (GOAL: 4-6)   WEIGHT: _____

4. DIP
(ALTERNATIVE: ASSISTED DIP OR SEATED DIP W/ MACHINE)

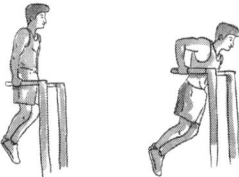

PREVIOUS BEST (WORKOUT 38)   REPS: _____   WEIGHT: _____

SET 1   REPS: _____   (GOAL: TO FAILURE)   WEIGHT: _____
SET 2   REPS: _____   (GOAL: TO FAILURE)   WEIGHT: _____
SET 3   REPS: _____   (GOAL: TO FAILURE)   WEIGHT: _____
SET 4 (OPTIONAL)   REPS: _____   (GOAL: TO FAILURE)   WEIGHT: _____

SUPERSETS DONE TODAY (CIRCLE):
1   2   3   4

TODAY'S WORKOUT INTENSITY:
_____ / 10

Workout 42: Back & Shoulders

1. ASSISTED PULL-UP
(ALTERNATIVE: PULL-UP OR TOWEL PULL)

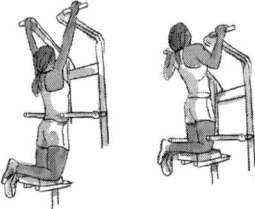

PREVIOUS BEST
(WORKOUT 38)   REPS: _____   WEIGHT: _____

SET 1   REPS: _____   (GOAL: 10-15)   WEIGHT: _____

SET 2   REPS: _____   (GOAL: 8-12)   WEIGHT: _____

SET 3   REPS: _____   (GOAL: 6-8)   WEIGHT: _____

SET 4   REPS: _____   (GOAL: 4-6)   WEIGHT: _____
(OPTIONAL)

2. T-BAR ROW
(ALTERNATIVE: UPPER BACK ROPE PULL)

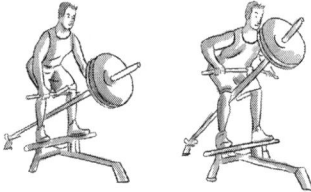

PREVIOUS BEST
(WORKOUT 38)   REPS: _____   WEIGHT: _____

SET 1   REPS: _____   (GOAL: 10-15)   WEIGHT: _____

SET 2   REPS: _____   (GOAL: 8-12)   WEIGHT: _____

SET 3   REPS: _____   (GOAL: 6-8)   WEIGHT: _____

SET 4   REPS: _____   (GOAL: 4-6)   WEIGHT: _____
(OPTIONAL)

3. LAT PULLDOWN

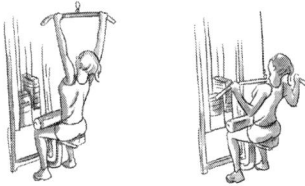

PREVIOUS BEST
(WORKOUT 38)   REPS: _____   WEIGHT: _____

SET 1   REPS: _____   (GOAL: 10-15)   WEIGHT: _____

SET 2   REPS: _____   (GOAL: 8-12)   WEIGHT: _____

SET 3   REPS: _____   (GOAL: 6-8)   WEIGHT: _____

SET 4   REPS: _____   (GOAL: 4-6)   WEIGHT: _____
(OPTIONAL)

4. CLOSE GRIP CABLE ROW
(ALTERNATIVE: PULL-UP OR LAT ROW)

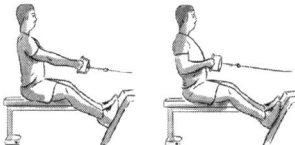

PREVIOUS BEST
(WORKOUT 38)   REPS: _____   WEIGHT: _____

SET 1   REPS: _____   (GOAL: 10-15)   WEIGHT: _____

SET 2   REPS: _____   (GOAL: 8-12)   WEIGHT: _____

SET 3   REPS: _____   (GOAL: 6-8)   WEIGHT: _____

SET 4   REPS: _____   (GOAL: 4-6)   WEIGHT: _____
(OPTIONAL)

AMOUNT OF CARDIO DONE TODAY:

Workout 42: Back & Shoulders

1. LATERAL DUMBBELL RAISE

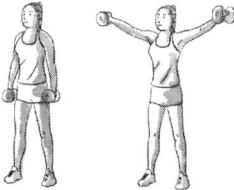

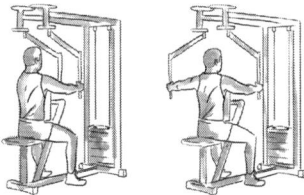

PREVIOUS BEST
(WORKOUT 36)   REPS: _____   WEIGHT: _____

SET 1   REPS: _____   (GOAL: 10-15)   WEIGHT: _____

SET 2   REPS: _____   (GOAL: 8-12)   WEIGHT: _____

SET 3   REPS: _____   (GOAL: 6-8)   WEIGHT: _____

SET 4   REPS: _____   (GOAL: 4-6)   WEIGHT: _____
(OPTIONAL)

2. FRONT DUMBBELL RAISE

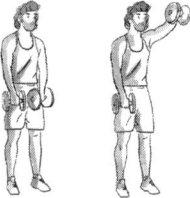

PREVIOUS BEST
(WORKOUT 33)   REPS: _____   WEIGHT: _____

SET 1   REPS: _____   (GOAL: 10-15)   WEIGHT: _____

SET 2   REPS: _____   (GOAL: 8-12)   WEIGHT: _____

SET 3   REPS: _____   (GOAL: 6-8)   WEIGHT: _____

SET 4   REPS: _____   (GOAL: 4-6)   WEIGHT: _____
(OPTIONAL)

3. REVERSE FLY

PREVIOUS BEST
(WORKOUT 36)   REPS: _____   WEIGHT: _____

SET 1   REPS: _____   (GOAL: 10-15)   WEIGHT: _____

SET 2   REPS: _____   (GOAL: 8-12)   WEIGHT: _____

SET 3   REPS: _____   (GOAL: 6-8)   WEIGHT: _____

SET 4   REPS: _____   (GOAL: 4-6)   WEIGHT: _____
(OPTIONAL)

4. SEATED DUMBBELL PRESS

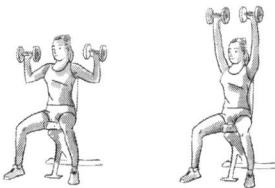

PREVIOUS BEST
(WORKOUT 33)   REPS: _____   WEIGHT: _____

SET 1   REPS: _____   (GOAL: 10-15)   WEIGHT: _____

SET 2   REPS: _____   (GOAL: 8-12)   WEIGHT: _____

SET 3   REPS: _____   (GOAL: 6-8)   WEIGHT: _____

SET 4   REPS: _____   (GOAL: 4-6)   WEIGHT: _____
(OPTIONAL)

SUPERSETS DONE TODAY (CIRCLE):

1   2   3   4

TODAY'S WORKOUT INTENSITY:

_____ / 10

Workout 43: Chest & Forearms

DATE _____

1. FLAT BENCH PRESS

(ALTERNATIVE: FLAT BENCH DUMBBELL PRESS)

PREVIOUS BEST
(WORKOUT 37)

REPS: _____   WEIGHT: _____

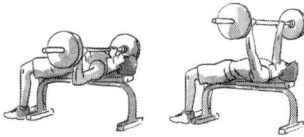

SET 1	REPS: _____	(GOAL: 10-15)	WEIGHT: _____
SET 2	REPS: _____	(GOAL: 8-12)	WEIGHT: _____
SET 3	REPS: _____	(GOAL: 6-8)	WEIGHT: _____
SET 4 (OPTIONAL)	REPS: _____	(GOAL: 4-6)	WEIGHT: _____

2. HIGH TO LOW CABLE FLY

PREVIOUS BEST
(WORKOUT 31)

REPS: _____   WEIGHT: _____

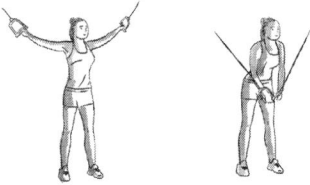

SET 1	REPS: _____	(GOAL: 10-15)	WEIGHT: _____
SET 2	REPS: _____	(GOAL: 8-12)	WEIGHT: _____
SET 3	REPS: _____	(GOAL: 6-8)	WEIGHT: _____
SET 4 (OPTIONAL)	REPS: _____	(GOAL: 4-6)	WEIGHT: _____

3. INCLINE BENCH PRESS

(ALTERNATIVE: INCLINE DUMBBELL PRESS)

PREVIOUS BEST
(WORKOUT 22)

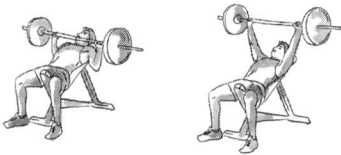

SET 1	REPS: _____	(GOAL: 10-15)	WEIGHT: _____
SET 2	REPS: _____	(GOAL: 8-12)	WEIGHT: _____
SET 3	REPS: _____	(GOAL: 6-8)	WEIGHT: _____
SET 4 (OPTIONAL)	REPS: _____	(GOAL: 4-6)	WEIGHT: _____

4. LOW TO HIGH CABLE FLY

PREVIOUS BEST
(WORKOUT 31)

REPS: _____   WEIGHT: _____

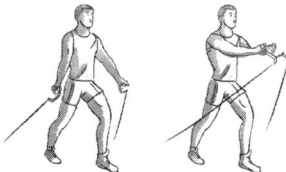

SET 1	REPS: _____	(GOAL: 10-15)	WEIGHT: _____
SET 2	REPS: _____	(GOAL: 8-12)	WEIGHT: _____
SET 3	REPS: _____	(GOAL: 6-8)	WEIGHT: _____
SET 4 (OPTIONAL)	REPS: _____	(GOAL: 4-6)	WEIGHT: _____

🏃 **AMOUNT OF CARDIO DONE TODAY:** _____

Workout 43: Chest & Forearms

5. DUMBBELL PULLOVER

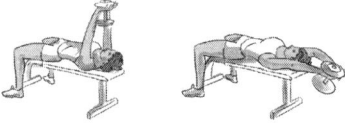

PREVIOUS BEST
(WORKOUT 17)

REPS: _____ WEIGHT: _____

SET 1	REPS: _____	(GOAL: 10-15)	WEIGHT: _____
SET 2	REPS: _____	(GOAL: 8-12)	WEIGHT: _____
SET 3	REPS: _____	(GOAL: 6-8)	WEIGHT: _____
SET 4 (OPTIONAL)	REPS: _____	(GOAL: 4-6)	WEIGHT: _____

1. REVERSE GRIP EZ BAR CURL

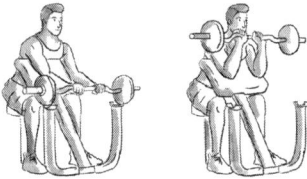

PREVIOUS BEST
(WORKOUT 28)

REPS: _____ WEIGHT: _____

SET 1	REPS: _____	(GOAL: 10-15)	WEIGHT: _____
SET 2	REPS: _____	(GOAL: 8-12)	WEIGHT: _____
SET 3	REPS: _____	(GOAL: 6-8)	WEIGHT: _____
SET 4 (OPTIONAL)	REPS: _____	(GOAL: 4-6)	WEIGHT: _____

2. BARBELL TWIST-UP

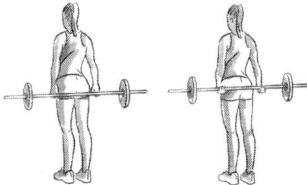

PREVIOUS BEST
(WORKOUT 28)

REPS: _____ WEIGHT: _____

SET 1	REPS: _____	(GOAL: 10-15)	WEIGHT: _____
SET 2	REPS: _____	(GOAL: 8-12)	WEIGHT: _____
SET 3	REPS: _____	(GOAL: 6-8)	WEIGHT: _____
SET 4 (OPTIONAL)	REPS: _____	(GOAL: 4-6)	WEIGHT: _____

SUPERSETS DONE TODAY (CIRCLE):
1   2   3   4

TODAY'S WORKOUT INTENSITY:
_____ / 10

Workout 44: Legs & Abs

DATE _____

1. LEG PRESS

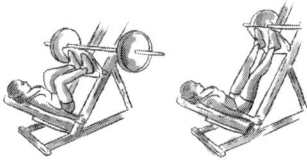

PREVIOUS BEST (WORKOUT 34)	REPS: _____	WEIGHT: _____
SET 1	REPS: _____ (GOAL: 10-15)	WEIGHT: _____
SET 2	REPS: _____ (GOAL: 8-12)	WEIGHT: _____
SET 3	REPS: _____ (GOAL: 6-8)	WEIGHT: _____
SET 4 (OPTIONAL)	REPS: _____ (GOAL: 4-6)	WEIGHT: _____

2. HACK SQUAT
(ALTERNATIVE: WEIGHTED LUNGE)

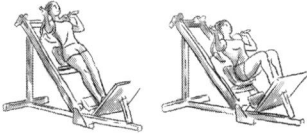

PREVIOUS BEST (WORKOUT 34)	REPS: _____	WEIGHT: _____
SET 1	REPS: _____ (GOAL: 10-15)	WEIGHT: _____
SET 2	REPS: _____ (GOAL: 8-12)	WEIGHT: _____
SET 3	REPS: _____ (GOAL: 6-8)	WEIGHT: _____
SET 4 (OPTIONAL)	REPS: _____ (GOAL: 4-6)	WEIGHT: _____

3. WEIGHTED LUNGE
(ALTERNATIVE: QUAD EXTENSION)

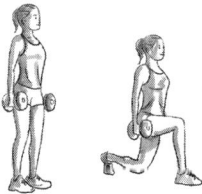

PREVIOUS BEST (WORKOUT 29)	REPS: _____	WEIGHT: _____
SET 1	REPS: _____ (GOAL: 10-15)	WEIGHT: _____
SET 2	REPS: _____ (GOAL: 8-12)	WEIGHT: _____
SET 3	REPS: _____ (GOAL: 6-8)	WEIGHT: _____
SET 4 (OPTIONAL)	REPS: _____ (GOAL: 4-6)	WEIGHT: _____

4. HAMSTRING EXTENSION

PREVIOUS BEST (WORKOUT 39)	REPS: _____	WEIGHT: _____
SET 1	REPS: _____ (GOAL: 10-15)	WEIGHT: _____
SET 2	REPS: _____ (GOAL: 8-12)	WEIGHT: _____
SET 3	REPS: _____ (GOAL: 6-8)	WEIGHT: _____
SET 4 (OPTIONAL)	REPS: _____ (GOAL: 4-6)	WEIGHT: _____

AMOUNT OF CARDIO DONE TODAY: _____

<u>Workout 44: Legs & Abs</u>

5. CALF RAISE
(ALTERNATIVE: SEATED CALF PRESS MACHINE)

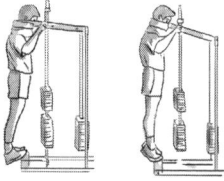

PREVIOUS BEST REPS: _____ WEIGHT: _____
(WORKOUT 39)

SET 1	REPS: _____	(GOAL: 10-15)	WEIGHT: _____
SET 2	REPS: _____	(GOAL: 8-12)	WEIGHT: _____
SET 3	REPS: _____	(GOAL: 6-8)	WEIGHT: _____
SET 4	REPS: _____	(GOAL: 4-6)	WEIGHT: _____
(OPTIONAL)			

1. KNEELING CABLE CRUNCH

PREVIOUS BEST REPS: _____ WEIGHT: _____
(WORKOUT 39)

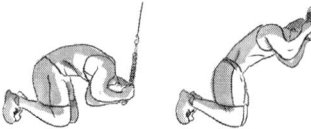

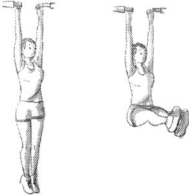

SET 1	REPS: _____	(GOAL: 10-20)	WEIGHT: _____
SET 2	REPS: _____	(GOAL: 10-20)	WEIGHT: _____
SET 3	REPS: _____	(GOAL: 10-20)	WEIGHT: _____

2. RUSSIAN TWIST

PREVIOUS BEST REPS: _____
(WORKOUT 31)

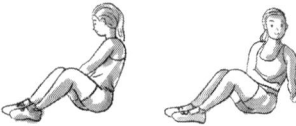

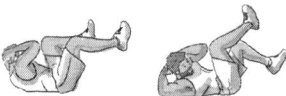

SET 1	REPS: _____	(GOAL: 10-20 EACH SIDE)
SET 2	REPS: _____	(GOAL: 10-20 EACH SIDE)
SET 3	REPS: _____	(GOAL: 10-20 EACH SIDE)

3. HANGING LEG LIFT

PREVIOUS BEST REPS: _____
(WORKOUT 39)

SET 1	REPS: _____	(GOAL: 10-20)
SET 2	REPS: _____	(GOAL: 10-20)
SET 3	REPS: _____	(GOAL: 10-20)

4. BICYCLE CRUNCH

PREVIOUS BEST REPS: _____
(WORKOUT 37)

SET 1	REPS: _____	(GOAL: 10-20 EACH SIDE)
SET 2	REPS: _____	(GOAL: 10-20 EACH SIDE)
SET 3	REPS: _____	(GOAL: 10-20 EACH SIDE)

SUPERSETS DONE TODAY (CIRCLE):

1   2   3   4

TODAY'S WORKOUT INTENSITY:

_____ / 10

Workout 45: Full Body Circuit

Rest for **15-20 seconds** between each exercise, then rest for **1-2 minutes** after completing the entire circuit. Complete the full circuit **a total of 4-5 times.**

1. RUN IN PLACE

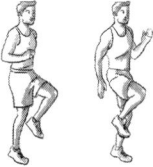

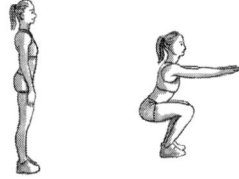

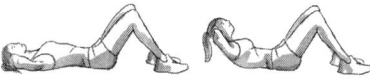

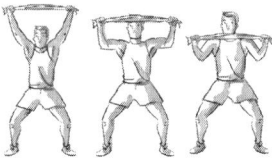

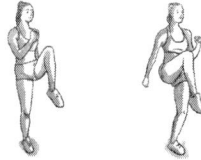

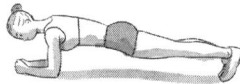

(Duration: 30 Seconds)

2. AIR SQUAT

(Duration: 30 Seconds)

3. CRUNCH

(Duration: 30 Seconds)

4. MOUNTAIN CLIMBER

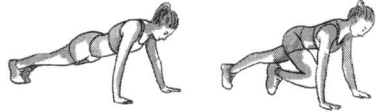

(Duration: 30 Seconds)

5. TOWEL PULL

(Duration: 30 Seconds)

6. HIGH KNEE

(Duration: 30 Seconds)

7. IN AND OUT PUSH-UP

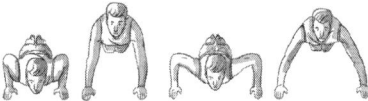

(Duration: 30 Seconds)

8. PLANK

(Duration: 30 Seconds)

TODAY'S WORKOUT INTENSITY:

_____ / 10

<u>Pro-Tip</u>

Notice if your supporting muscles are too weak for a movement.

If you notice you're shifting your body in weird ways and not maintaining perfect form during all points of each exercise, you are likely making this large mistake:

The weight you're using is enough for your main muscle (e.g. chest) but too heavy for your underdeveloped supporting muscle (e.g. triceps).

By knowing exactly which muscles are used in each movement, you'll be able to identify the 'weakest link' and improve the strength of that muscle by very intensely mentally focusing on its performance through each rep of your movement.

If you notice this is happening with you, an effective remedy is to add an extra day working that weak secondary muscle specifically (e.g. working triceps out 2x a week).

Alternatively, you can add 3-4 extra sets of that muscle at the end of each workout (even of different body parts) to catch it up.

Workout 46: Chest & Biceps

DATE _____

1. FLAT BENCH PRESS

(ALTERNATIVE: FLAT BENCH DUMBBELL PRESS)

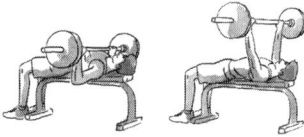

PREVIOUS BEST (WORKOUT 43)   REPS: _____   WEIGHT: _____

SET 1	REPS: _____	(GOAL: 10-15)	WEIGHT: _____
SET 2	REPS: _____	(GOAL: 8-12)	WEIGHT: _____
SET 3	REPS: _____	(GOAL: 6-8)	WEIGHT: _____
SET 4 (OPTIONAL)	REPS: _____	(GOAL: 4-6)	WEIGHT: _____

2. INCLINE BENCH PRESS

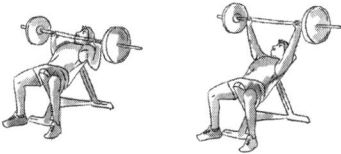

PREVIOUS BEST (WORKOUT 43)   REPS: _____   WEIGHT: _____

SET 1	REPS: _____	(GOAL: 10-15)	WEIGHT: _____
SET 2	REPS: _____	(GOAL: 8-12)	WEIGHT: _____
SET 3	REPS: _____	(GOAL: 6-8)	WEIGHT: _____
SET 4 (OPTIONAL)	REPS: _____	(GOAL: 4-6)	WEIGHT: _____

3. HIGH TO LOW CABLE FLY

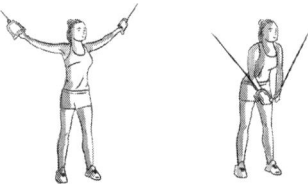

PREVIOUS BEST (WORKOUT 43)   REPS: _____   WEIGHT: _____

SET 1	REPS: _____	(GOAL: 10-15)	WEIGHT: _____
SET 2	REPS: _____	(GOAL: 8-12)	WEIGHT: _____
SET 3	REPS: _____	(GOAL: 6-8)	WEIGHT: _____
SET 4 (OPTIONAL)	REPS: _____	(GOAL: 4-6)	WEIGHT: _____

4. FLAT BENCH DUMBBELL FLY

(ALTERNATIVE: CHEST FLY W/ MACHINE)

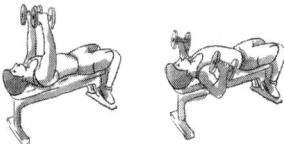

PREVIOUS BEST (WORKOUT 37)   REPS: _____   WEIGHT: _____

SET 1	REPS: _____	(GOAL: 10-15)	WEIGHT: _____
SET 2	REPS: _____	(GOAL: 8-12)	WEIGHT: _____
SET 3	REPS: _____	(GOAL: 6-8)	WEIGHT: _____
SET 4 (OPTIONAL)	REPS: _____	(GOAL: 4-6)	WEIGHT: _____

AMOUNT OF CARDIO DONE TODAY: _____

Workout 46: Chest & Biceps

1. PREACHER CURL
(ALTERNATIVE: SEATED DUMBBELL CURL)

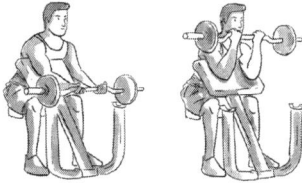

PREVIOUS BEST
(WORKOUT 41)

REPS: _____   WEIGHT: _____

SET 1	REPS: _____ (GOAL: 10-15)	WEIGHT: _____
SET 2	REPS: _____ (GOAL: 8-12)	WEIGHT: _____
SET 3	REPS: _____ (GOAL: 6-8)	WEIGHT: _____
SET 4 (OPTIONAL)	REPS: _____ (GOAL: 4-6)	WEIGHT: _____

2. DUMBBELL HAMMER CURL

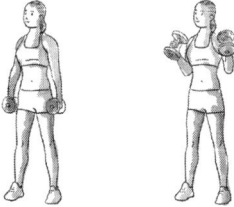

PREVIOUS BEST
(WORKOUT 22)

REPS: _____   WEIGHT: _____

SET 1	REPS: _____ (GOAL: 10-15)	WEIGHT: _____
SET 2	REPS: _____ (GOAL: 8-12)	WEIGHT: _____
SET 3	REPS: _____ (GOAL: 6-8)	WEIGHT: _____
SET 4 (OPTIONAL)	REPS: _____ (GOAL: 4-6)	WEIGHT: _____

3. CONCENTRATION CURL

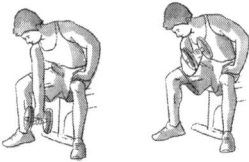

PREVIOUS BEST
(WORKOUT 36)

REPS: _____   WEIGHT: _____

SET 1	REPS: _____ (GOAL: 10-15)	WEIGHT: _____
SET 2	REPS: _____ (GOAL: 8-12)	WEIGHT: _____
SET 3	REPS: _____ (GOAL: 6-8)	WEIGHT: _____
SET 4 (OPTIONAL)	REPS: _____ (GOAL: 4-6)	WEIGHT: _____

4. OVERHEAD CABLE CURL

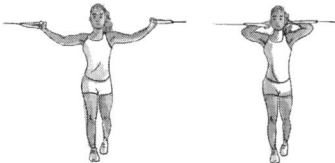

PREVIOUS BEST
(WORKOUT 36)

REPS: _____   WEIGHT: _____

SET 1	REPS: _____ (GOAL: 10-15)	WEIGHT: _____
SET 2	REPS: _____ (GOAL: 8-12)	WEIGHT: _____
SET 3	REPS: _____ (GOAL: 6-8)	WEIGHT: _____
SET 4 (OPTIONAL)	REPS: _____ (GOAL: 4-6)	WEIGHT: _____

SUPERSETS DONE TODAY (CIRCLE):
1   2   3   4

TODAY'S WORKOUT INTENSITY:
_____ / 10

Workout 47: Back & Triceps

DATE _____

1. BENT OVER DUMBBELL ROW

(ALTERNATIVE: ASSISTED PULL-UP
OR TOWEL PULL)

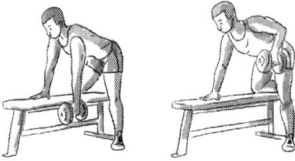

PREVIOUS BEST
(WORKOUT 27)

REPS: _____   WEIGHT: _____

SET 1	REPS: _____	(GOAL: 10-15)	WEIGHT: _____
SET 2	REPS: _____	(GOAL: 8-12)	WEIGHT: _____
SET 3	REPS: _____	(GOAL: 6-8)	WEIGHT: _____
SET 4 (OPTIONAL)	REPS: _____	(GOAL: 4-6)	WEIGHT: _____

2. UPPER BACK ROPE PULL

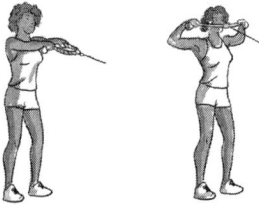

PREVIOUS BEST
(WORKOUT 21)

REPS: _____   WEIGHT: _____

SET 1	REPS: _____	(GOAL: 10-15)	WEIGHT: _____
SET 2	REPS: _____	(GOAL: 8-12)	WEIGHT: _____
SET 3	REPS: _____	(GOAL: 6-8)	WEIGHT: _____
SET 4 (OPTIONAL)	REPS: _____	(GOAL: 4-6)	WEIGHT: _____

3. STRAIGHT ARM PULLDOWN

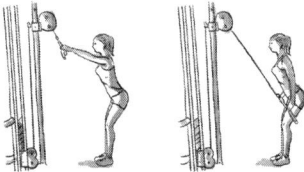

PREVIOUS BEST
(WORKOUT 32)

REPS: _____   WEIGHT: _____

SET 1	REPS: _____	(GOAL: 10-15)	WEIGHT: _____
SET 2	REPS: _____	(GOAL: 8-12)	WEIGHT: _____
SET 3	REPS: _____	(GOAL: 6-8)	WEIGHT: _____
SET 4 (OPTIONAL)	REPS: _____	(GOAL: 4-6)	WEIGHT: _____

4. CLOSE GRIP CABLE ROW

(ALTERNATIVE: PULL-UP OR LAT ROW)

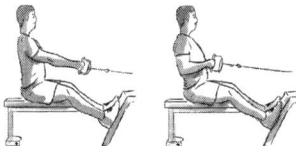

PREVIOUS BEST
(WORKOUT 42)

REPS: _____   WEIGHT: _____

SET 1	REPS: _____	(GOAL: 10-15)	WEIGHT: _____
SET 2	REPS: _____	(GOAL: 8-12)	WEIGHT: _____
SET 3	REPS: _____	(GOAL: 6-8)	WEIGHT: _____
SET 4 (OPTIONAL)	REPS: _____	(GOAL: 4-6)	WEIGHT: _____

AMOUNT OF CARDIO DONE TODAY: _____

Workout 47: Back & Triceps

1. OVERHEAD DUMBBELL EXTENSION

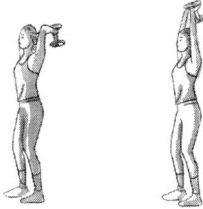

PREVIOUS BEST (WORKOUT 41)	REPS: _____	WEIGHT: _____
SET 1	REPS: _____ (GOAL: 10-15)	WEIGHT: _____
SET 2	REPS: _____ (GOAL: 8-12)	WEIGHT: _____
SET 3	REPS: _____ (GOAL: 6-8)	WEIGHT: _____
SET 4 (OPTIONAL)	REPS: _____ (GOAL: 4-6)	WEIGHT: _____

2. STRAIGHT BAR PULLDOWN

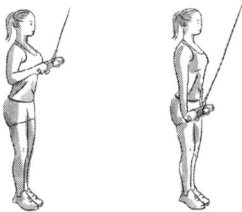

PREVIOUS BEST (WORKOUT 27)	REPS: _____	WEIGHT: _____
SET 1	REPS: _____ (GOAL: 10-15)	WEIGHT: _____
SET 2	REPS: _____ (GOAL: 8-12)	WEIGHT: _____
SET 3	REPS: _____ (GOAL: 6-8)	WEIGHT: _____
SET 4 (OPTIONAL)	REPS: _____ (GOAL: 4-6)	WEIGHT: _____

3. ROPE PULLDOWN

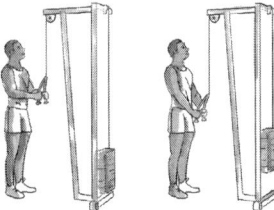

PREVIOUS BEST (WORKOUT 41)	REPS: _____	WEIGHT: _____
SET 1	REPS: _____ (GOAL: 10-15)	WEIGHT: _____
SET 2	REPS: _____ (GOAL: 8-12)	WEIGHT: _____
SET 3	REPS: _____ (GOAL: 6-8)	WEIGHT: _____
SET 4 (OPTIONAL)	REPS: _____ (GOAL: 4-6)	WEIGHT: _____

4. DIAMOND PUSH-UP

(ALTERNATIVE: ASSISTED DIP OR SEATED DIP W/ MACHINE)

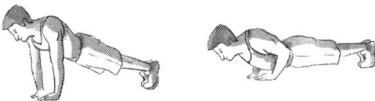

PREVIOUS BEST (WORKOUT 27)	REPS: _____
SET 1	REPS: _____ (GOAL: TO FAILURE)
SET 2	REPS: _____ (GOAL: TO FAILURE)
SET 3	REPS: _____ (GOAL: TO FAILURE)
SET 4 (OPTIONAL)	REPS: _____ (GOAL: TO FAILURE)

SUPERSETS DONE TODAY (CIRCLE):

1   2   3   4

TODAY'S WORKOUT INTENSITY:

_____ / 10

Workout 48: Shoulders & Forearms

DATE _____

1. BARBELL RAISE

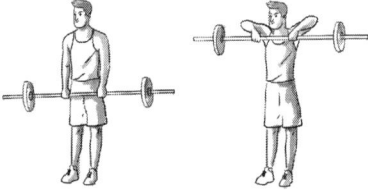

PREVIOUS BEST (WORKOUT 36)   REPS: _____   WEIGHT: _____

SET 1	REPS: _____ (GOAL: 10-15)	WEIGHT: _____
SET 2	REPS: _____ (GOAL: 8-12)	WEIGHT: _____
SET 3	REPS: _____ (GOAL: 6-8)	WEIGHT: _____
SET 4 (OPTIONAL)	REPS: _____ (GOAL: 4-6)	WEIGHT: _____

2. LATERAL DUMBBELL RAISE

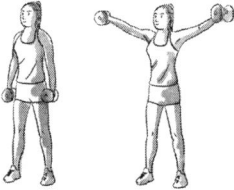

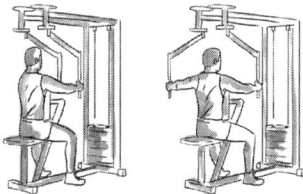

PREVIOUS BEST (WORKOUT 42)   REPS: _____   WEIGHT: _____

SET 1	REPS: _____ (GOAL: 10-15)	WEIGHT: _____
SET 2	REPS: _____ (GOAL: 8-12)	WEIGHT: _____
SET 3	REPS: _____ (GOAL: 6-8)	WEIGHT: _____
SET 4 (OPTIONAL)	REPS: _____ (GOAL: 4-6)	WEIGHT: _____

3. REVERSE FLY

PREVIOUS BEST (WORKOUT 42)   REPS: _____   WEIGHT: _____

SET 1	REPS: _____ (GOAL: 10-15)	WEIGHT: _____
SET 2	REPS: _____ (GOAL: 8-12)	WEIGHT: _____
SET 3	REPS: _____ (GOAL: 6-8)	WEIGHT: _____
SET 4 (OPTIONAL)	REPS: _____ (GOAL: 4-6)	WEIGHT: _____

4. ARNOLD DUMBBELL PRESS

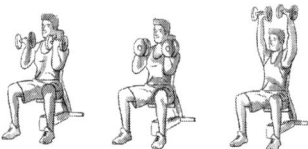

PREVIOUS BEST (WORKOUT 36)   REPS: _____   WEIGHT: _____

SET 1	REPS: _____ (GOAL: 10-15)	WEIGHT: _____
SET 2	REPS: _____ (GOAL: 8-12)	WEIGHT: _____
SET 3	REPS: _____ (GOAL: 6-8)	WEIGHT: _____
SET 4 (OPTIONAL)	REPS: _____ (GOAL: 4-6)	WEIGHT: _____

AMOUNT OF CARDIO DONE TODAY: _____

Workout 48: Shoulders & Forearms

5. SHRUG

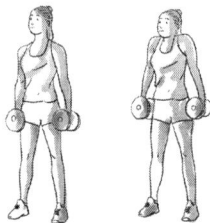

	PREVIOUS BEST (WORKOUT 18)	REPS: _____		WEIGHT: _____
	SET 1	REPS: _____	(GOAL: 10-15)	WEIGHT: _____
	SET 2	REPS: _____	(GOAL: 8-12)	WEIGHT: _____
	SET 3	REPS: _____	(GOAL: 6-8)	WEIGHT: _____
	SET 4 (OPTIONAL)	REPS: _____	(GOAL: 4-6)	WEIGHT: _____

1. REVERSE GRIP EZ BAR CURL
(ALTERNATIVE: FARMER'S WALK)

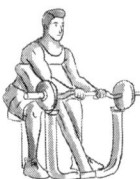

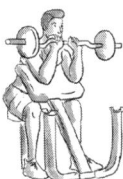

	PREVIOUS BEST (WORKOUT 43)	REPS: _____		WEIGHT: _____
	SET 1	REPS: _____	(GOAL: 10-15)	WEIGHT: _____
	SET 2	REPS: _____	(GOAL: 8-12)	WEIGHT: _____
	SET 3	REPS: _____	(GOAL: 6-8)	WEIGHT: _____
	SET 4 (OPTIONAL)	REPS: _____	(GOAL: 4-6)	WEIGHT: _____

2. BARBELL TWIST-UP
(ALTERNATIVE: PULL-UP BAR HANG)

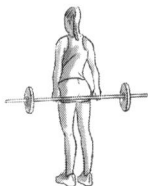

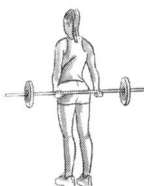

	PREVIOUS BEST (WORKOUT 43)	REPS: _____		WEIGHT: _____
	SET 1	REPS: _____	(GOAL: 10-15)	WEIGHT: _____
	SET 2	REPS: _____	(GOAL: 8-12)	WEIGHT: _____
	SET 3	REPS: _____	(GOAL: 6-8)	WEIGHT: _____
	SET 4 (OPTIONAL)	REPS: _____	(GOAL: 4-6)	WEIGHT: _____

SUPERSETS DONE TODAY (CIRCLE):
1   2   3   4

TODAY'S WORKOUT INTENSITY:
_____ / 10

EXERCISE
GUIDE
https://HabitNest.link/lifting49

Workout 49: Legs & Abs

DATE _____

1. DEADLIFT
(ALTERNATIVE: LEG PRESS)

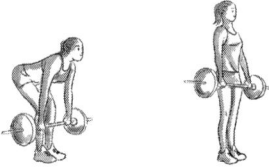

PREVIOUS BEST (WORKOUT 39)   REPS: _____   WEIGHT: _____

SET 1   REPS: _____ (GOAL: 10-15)   WEIGHT: _____
SET 2   REPS: _____ (GOAL: 8-12)   WEIGHT: _____
SET 3   REPS: _____ (GOAL: 6-8)   WEIGHT: _____
SET 4 (OPTIONAL)   REPS: _____ (GOAL: 4-6)   WEIGHT: _____

2. BARBELL SQUAT
(ALTERNATIVE: HACK SQUAT)

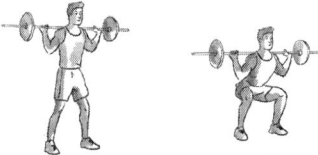

PREVIOUS BEST (WORKOUT 39)   REPS: _____   WEIGHT: _____

SET 1   REPS: _____ (GOAL: 10-15)   WEIGHT: _____
SET 2   REPS: _____ (GOAL: 8-12)   WEIGHT: _____
SET 3   REPS: _____ (GOAL: 6-8)   WEIGHT: _____
SET 4 (OPTIONAL)   REPS: _____ (GOAL: 4-6)   WEIGHT: _____

3. QUAD EXTENSION

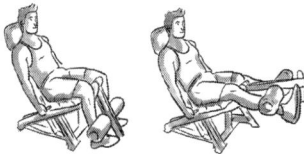

PREVIOUS BEST (WORKOUT 39)   REPS: _____   WEIGHT: _____

SET 1   REPS: _____ (GOAL: 10-15)   WEIGHT: _____
SET 2   REPS: _____ (GOAL: 8-12)   WEIGHT: _____
SET 3   REPS: _____ (GOAL: 6-8)   WEIGHT: _____
SET 4 (OPTIONAL)   REPS: _____ (GOAL: 4-6)   WEIGHT: _____

4. HAMSTRING EXTENSION

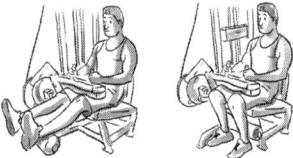

PREVIOUS BEST (WORKOUT 44)   REPS: _____   WEIGHT: _____

SET 1   REPS: _____ (GOAL: 10-15)   WEIGHT: _____
SET 2   REPS: _____ (GOAL: 8-12)   WEIGHT: _____
SET 3   REPS: _____ (GOAL: 6-8)   WEIGHT: _____
SET 4 (OPTIONAL)   REPS: _____ (GOAL: 4-6)   WEIGHT: _____

AMOUNT OF CARDIO DONE TODAY: _____

Workout 49: Legs & Abs

5. CALF RAISE
(ALTERNATIVE: SEATED CALF PRESS MACHINE)

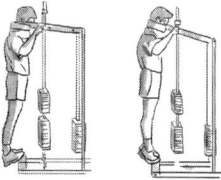

PREVIOUS BEST
(WORKOUT 44) REPS: _____   WEIGHT: _____

SET 1 REPS: _____ (GOAL: 10-15)   WEIGHT: _____

SET 2 REPS: _____ (GOAL: 8-12)   WEIGHT: _____

SET 3 REPS: _____ (GOAL: 6-8)   WEIGHT: _____

SET 4 REPS: _____ (GOAL: 4-6)   WEIGHT: _____
(OPTIONAL)

1. KNEELING CABLE CRUNCH

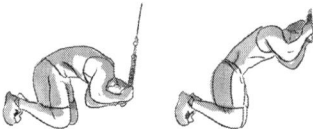

PREVIOUS BEST
(WORKOUT 44) REPS: _____   WEIGHT: _____

SET 1 REPS: _____ (GOAL: 10-20)   WEIGHT: _____

SET 2 REPS: _____ (GOAL: 10-20)   WEIGHT: _____

SET 3 REPS: _____ (GOAL: 10-20)   WEIGHT: _____

2. LEG LIFT

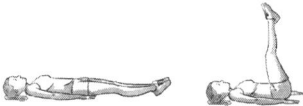

PREVIOUS BEST
(WORKOUT 34) REPS: _____

SET 1 REPS: _____ (GOAL: 10-20)

SET 2 REPS: _____ (GOAL:10-20)

SET 3 REPS: _____ (GOAL: 10-20)

3. STARFISH CRUNCH

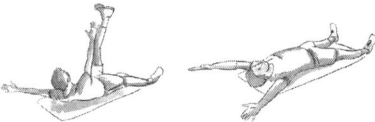

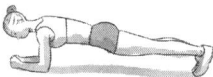

PREVIOUS BEST
(WORKOUT 39) REPS: _____

SET 1 REPS: _____ (GOAL: 10-20 EACH SIDE)

SET 2 REPS: _____ (GOAL: 10-20 EACH SIDE)

SET 3 REPS: _____ (GOAL: 10-20 EACH SIDE)

4. PLANK

PREVIOUS BEST
(WORKOUT 39) TIME: _____

SET 1 TIME: _____ (GOAL: 45-90 SECONDS)

SET 2 TIME: _____ (GOAL: 45-90 SECONDS)

SET 3 TIME: _____ (GOAL: 45-90 SECONDS)

SUPERSETS DONE TODAY (CIRCLE):

1   2   3   4

TODAY'S WORKOUT INTENSITY:

_____ / 10

Workout 50: Full Body Circuit

*Rest for **15-20 seconds** between each exercise, then rest for **1-2 minutes** after completing the entire circuit. Complete the full circuit **a total of 4-5 times.***

1. JUMPING JACK

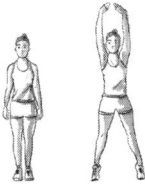

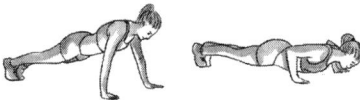

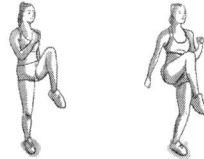

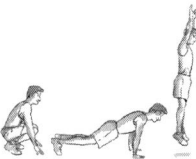

(Duration: 30 Seconds)

2. ALTERNATING LUNGE

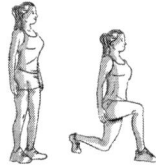

(Duration: 30 Seconds)

3. STARFISH CRUNCH

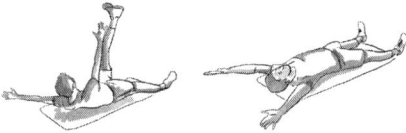

(Duration: 30 Seconds)

4. TOWEL SNATCH

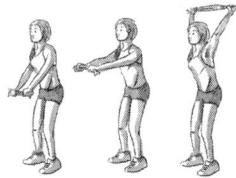

(Duration: 30 Seconds)

5. PUSH-UP

(Duration: 30 Seconds)

6. HIGH KNEE

(Duration: 30 Seconds)

7. BURPEE

(Duration: 30 Seconds)

8. BICYCLE CRUNCH

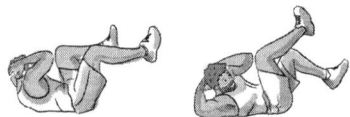

(Duration: 30 Seconds)

TODAY'S WORKOUT INTENSITY:
_____ / 10

<u>Check-In</u> ⊘

How far am I from where I wanted to be when I started this journal?

_____

_____

_____

_____

What do I think I need to do for the next few weeks to reach my initial goal by the end of the journal?

_____

_____

_____

_____

Which parts of my body am I noticing significant strength gains in? Which ones are still lacking?

_____

_____

_____

_____

_____

Bonus Challenge

> *Going forward, complete four dropsets in each workout.*

Dropsets are a fantastic way to push a muscle to a much further limit than you normally do during a workout.

A dropset consists of doing a set normally, then immediately dropping the weight by 25-50% and continuing the movement without rest to get extra reps in.

To take your workouts to the next level, on the last, fourth set of an exercise, perform a dropset. This only takes ~30 seconds or so each to do but will bring about an unforeseen level of intensity for that muscle as you're truly pushing it to its limit.

If you've previously taken on the other workout challenges, you can do this in addition to them. Simply choose four of the eight exercises each day to add a dropset at the end of.

(Optional)
I will complete a dropset at the end of four different exercises during my next workout.

_____   _____
Signature   Date

Workout 51: Back & Abs

DATE _____

1. ASSISTED PULL-UP
(ALTERNATIVE: PULL-UP OR TOWEL PULL)

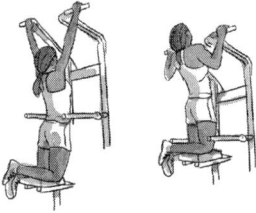

PREVIOUS BEST (WORKOUT 42) REPS: _____   WEIGHT: _____

SET 1 REPS: _____ (GOAL: 10-15)   WEIGHT: _____
SET 2 REPS: _____ (GOAL: 8-12)   WEIGHT: _____
SET 3 REPS: _____ (GOAL: 6-8)   WEIGHT: _____
SET 4 (OPTIONAL) REPS: _____ (GOAL: 4-6)   WEIGHT: _____

2. T-BAR ROW
(ALTERNATIVE: UPPER BACK ROPE PULL)

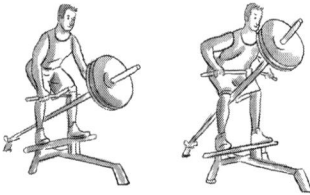

PREVIOUS BEST (WORKOUT 42) REPS: _____   WEIGHT: _____

SET 1 REPS: _____ (GOAL: 10-15)   WEIGHT: _____
SET 2 REPS: _____ (GOAL: 8-12)   WEIGHT: _____
SET 3 REPS: _____ (GOAL: 6-8)   WEIGHT: _____
SET 4 (OPTIONAL) REPS: _____ (GOAL: 4-6)   WEIGHT: _____

3. LAT PULLDOWN

PREVIOUS BEST (WORKOUT 42) REPS: _____   WEIGHT: _____

SET 1 REPS: _____ (GOAL: 10-15)   WEIGHT: _____
SET 2 REPS: _____ (GOAL: 8-12)   WEIGHT: _____
SET 3 REPS: _____ (GOAL: 6-8)   WEIGHT: _____
SET 4 (OPTIONAL) REPS: _____ (GOAL: 4-6)   WEIGHT: _____

4. CLOSE GRIP CABLE ROW
(ALTERNATIVE: PULL-UP OR LAT ROW)

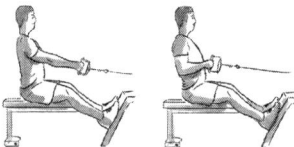

PREVIOUS BEST (WORKOUT 47) REPS: _____   WEIGHT: _____

SET 1 REPS: _____ (GOAL: 10-15)   WEIGHT: _____
SET 2 REPS: _____ (GOAL: 8-12)   WEIGHT: _____
SET 3 REPS: _____ (GOAL: 6-8)   WEIGHT: _____
SET 4 (OPTIONAL) REPS: _____ (GOAL: 4-6)   WEIGHT: _____

AMOUNT OF CARDIO DONE TODAY: _____

Workout 51: Back & Abs

5. UPPER BACK ROPE PULL

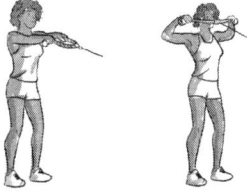

PREVIOUS BEST (WORKOUT 47)	REPS: _____		WEIGHT: _____
SET 1	REPS: _____	(GOAL: 10-15)	WEIGHT: _____
SET 2	REPS: _____	(GOAL: 8-12)	WEIGHT: _____
SET 3	REPS: _____	(GOAL: 6-8)	WEIGHT: _____
SET 4 (OPTIONAL)	REPS: _____	(GOAL: 4-6)	WEIGHT: _____

1. KNEELING CABLE CRUNCH

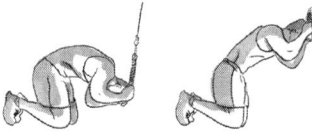

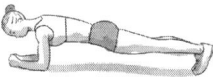

PREVIOUS BEST (WORKOUT 49)	REPS: _____		WEIGHT: _____
SET 1	REPS: _____	(GOAL: 10-20)	WEIGHT: _____
SET 2	REPS: _____	(GOAL: 10-20)	WEIGHT: _____
SET 3	REPS: _____	(GOAL: 10-20)	WEIGHT: _____

2. HANGING LEG LIFT

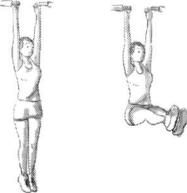

PREVIOUS BEST (WORKOUT 44)	REPS: _____	
SET 1	REPS: _____	(GOAL: 10-20)
SET 2	REPS: _____	(GOAL: 10-20)
SET 3	REPS: _____	(GOAL: 10-20)

3. BICYCLE CRUNCH

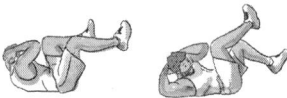

PREVIOUS BEST (WORKOUT 44)	REPS: _____	
SET 1	REPS: _____	(GOAL: 10-20 EACH SIDE)
SET 2	REPS: _____	(GOAL: 10-20 EACH SIDE)
SET 3	REPS: _____	(GOAL: 10-20 EACH SIDE)

4. PLANK

PREVIOUS BEST (WORKOUT 49)	TIME: _____	
SET 1	TIME: _____	(GOAL: 45-90 SECONDS)
SET 2	TIME: _____	(GOAL: 45-90 SECONDS)
SET 3	TIME: _____	(GOAL: 45-90 SECONDS)

SUPERSETS DONE TODAY (CIRCLE):

1   2   3   4

TODAY'S WORKOUT INTENSITY:

_____ / 10

<u>Workout 52: Chest</u> & Biceps

1. FLAT BENCH PRESS

(ALTERNATIVE: FLAT BENCH DUMBBELL PRESS)

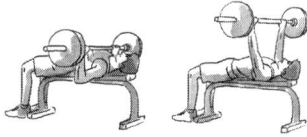

PREVIOUS BEST (WORKOUT 46)	REPS: _____	WEIGHT: _____
SET 1	REPS: _____ (GOAL: 10-15)	WEIGHT: _____
SET 2	REPS: _____ (GOAL: 8-12)	WEIGHT: _____
SET 3	REPS: _____ (GOAL: 6-8)	WEIGHT: _____
SET 4 (OPTIONAL)	REPS: _____ (GOAL: 4-6)	WEIGHT: _____

2. INCLINE BENCH PRESS

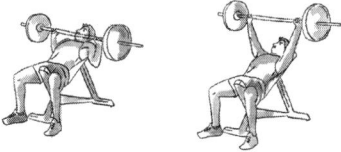

PREVIOUS BEST (WORKOUT 46)	REPS: _____	WEIGHT: _____
SET 1	REPS: _____ (GOAL: 10-15)	WEIGHT: _____
SET 2	REPS: _____ (GOAL: 8-12)	WEIGHT: _____
SET 3	REPS: _____ (GOAL: 6-8)	WEIGHT: _____
SET 4 (OPTIONAL)	REPS: _____ (GOAL: 4-6)	WEIGHT: _____

3. HIGH TO LOW CABLE FLY

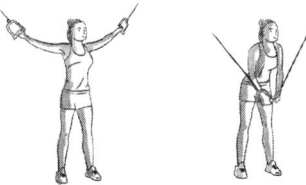

PREVIOUS BEST (WORKOUT 46)	REPS: _____	WEIGHT: _____
SET 1	REPS: _____ (GOAL: 10-15)	WEIGHT: _____
SET 2	REPS: _____ (GOAL: 8-12)	WEIGHT: _____
SET 3	REPS: _____ (GOAL: 6-8)	WEIGHT: _____
SET 4 (OPTIONAL)	REPS: _____ (GOAL: 4-6)	WEIGHT: _____

4. FLAT BENCH DUMBBELL FLY

(ALTERNATIVE: CHEST FLY W/ MACHINE)

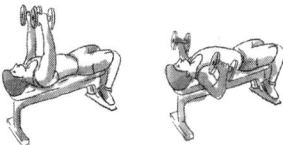

PREVIOUS BEST (WORKOUT 46)	REPS: _____	WEIGHT: _____
SET 1	REPS: _____ (GOAL: 10-15)	WEIGHT: _____
SET 2	REPS: _____ (GOAL: 8-12)	WEIGHT: _____
SET 3	REPS: _____ (GOAL: 6-8)	WEIGHT: _____
SET 4 (OPTIONAL)	REPS: _____ (GOAL: 4-6)	WEIGHT: _____

AMOUNT OF CARDIO DONE TODAY:
_____

176

Workout 52: Chest & Biceps

1. PREACHER CURL

(ALTERNATIVE: SEATED DUMBBELL CURL)

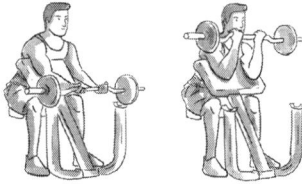

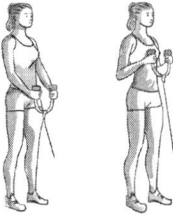

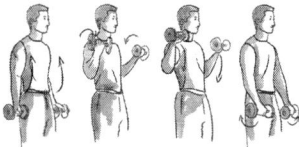

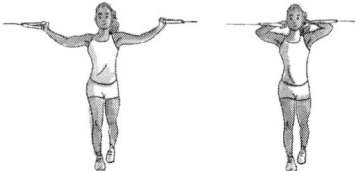

PREVIOUS BEST [WORKOUT 46]	REPS: _____	WEIGHT: _____
SET 1	REPS: _____ (GOAL: 10-15)	WEIGHT: _____
SET 2	REPS: _____ (GOAL: 8-12)	WEIGHT: _____
SET 3	REPS: _____ (GOAL: 6-8)	WEIGHT: _____
SET 4 (OPTIONAL)	REPS: _____ (GOAL: 4-6)	WEIGHT: _____

2. ROPE HAMMER CURL

PREVIOUS BEST [WORKOUT 32]	REPS: _____	WEIGHT: _____
SET 1	REPS: _____ (GOAL: 10-15)	WEIGHT: _____
SET 2	REPS: _____ (GOAL: 8-12)	WEIGHT: _____
SET 3	REPS: _____ (GOAL: 6-8)	WEIGHT: _____
SET 4 (OPTIONAL)	REPS: _____ (GOAL: 4-6)	WEIGHT: _____

3. ZOTTMAN CURL

PREVIOUS BEST [WORKOUT 41]	REPS: _____	WEIGHT: _____
SET 1	REPS: _____ (GOAL: 10-15)	WEIGHT: _____
SET 2	REPS: _____ (GOAL: 8-12)	WEIGHT: _____
SET 3	REPS: _____ (GOAL: 6-8)	WEIGHT: _____
SET 4 (OPTIONAL)	REPS: _____ (GOAL: 4-6)	WEIGHT: _____

4. OVERHEAD CABLE CURL

PREVIOUS BEST [WORKOUT 46]	REPS: _____	WEIGHT: _____
SET 1	REPS: _____ (GOAL: 10-15)	WEIGHT: _____
SET 2	REPS: _____ (GOAL: 8-12)	WEIGHT: _____
SET 3	REPS: _____ (GOAL: 6-8)	WEIGHT: _____
SET 4 (OPTIONAL)	REPS: _____ (GOAL: 4-6)	WEIGHT: _____

SUPERSETS DONE TODAY (CIRCLE):

1   2   3   4

TODAY'S WORKOUT INTENSITY:

_____ / 10

Workout 53: Shoulders & Triceps

1. LATERAL DUMBBELL RAISE

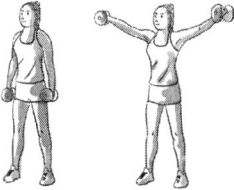

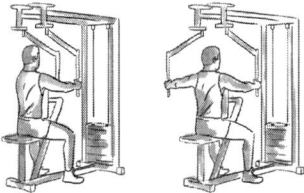

PREVIOUS BEST
(WORKOUT 48)   REPS: _____   WEIGHT: _____

SET 1   REPS: _____   (GOAL: 10-15)   WEIGHT: _____

SET 2   REPS: _____   (GOAL: 8-12)   WEIGHT: _____

SET 3   REPS: _____   (GOAL: 6-8)   WEIGHT: _____

SET 4   REPS: _____   (GOAL: 4-6)   WEIGHT: _____
(OPTIONAL)

2. FRONT DUMBBELL RAISE

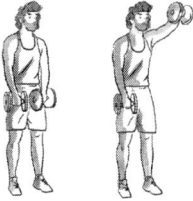

PREVIOUS BEST
(WORKOUT 42)   REPS: _____   WEIGHT: _____

SET 1   REPS: _____   (GOAL: 10-15)   WEIGHT: _____

SET 2   REPS: _____   (GOAL: 8-12)   WEIGHT: _____

SET 3   REPS: _____   (GOAL: 6-8)   WEIGHT: _____

SET 4   REPS: _____   (GOAL: 4-6)   WEIGHT: _____
(OPTIONAL)

3. REVERSE FLY

PREVIOUS BEST
(WORKOUT 48)   REPS: _____   WEIGHT: _____

SET 1   REPS: _____   (GOAL: 10-15)   WEIGHT: _____

SET 2   REPS: _____   (GOAL: 8-12)   WEIGHT: _____

SET 3   REPS: _____   (GOAL: 6-8)   WEIGHT: _____

SET 4   REPS: _____   (GOAL: 4-6)   WEIGHT: _____
(OPTIONAL)

4. SEATED DUMBBELL PRESS

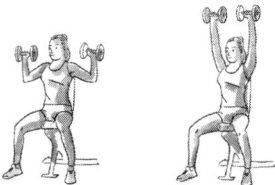

PREVIOUS BEST
(WORKOUT 42)   REPS: _____   WEIGHT: _____

SET 1   REPS: _____   (GOAL: 10-15)   WEIGHT: _____

SET 2   REPS: _____   (GOAL: 8-12)   WEIGHT: _____

SET 3   REPS: _____   (GOAL: 6-8)   WEIGHT: _____

SET 4   REPS: _____   (GOAL: 4-6)   WEIGHT: _____
(OPTIONAL)

🏃 AMOUNT OF CARDIO DONE TODAY:
_____

Workout 53: Shoulders & Triceps

1. SKULL CRUSHER

(ALTERNATIVE: CLOSE GRIP BENCH PRESS OR
DUMBBELL PULLOVER)

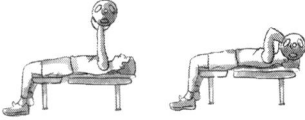

PREVIOUS BEST
(WORKOUT 41)

REPS: _____   WEIGHT: _____

SET 1 REPS: _____ (GOAL: 10-15) WEIGHT: _____

SET 2 REPS: _____ (GOAL: 8-12) WEIGHT: _____

SET 3 REPS: _____ (GOAL: 6-8) WEIGHT: _____

SET 4 REPS: _____ (GOAL: 4-6) WEIGHT: _____
(OPTIONAL)

2. OVERHEAD DUMBBELL EXTENSION

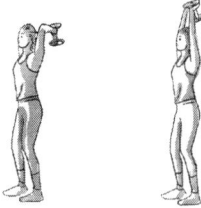

PREVIOUS BEST
(WORKOUT 47)

REPS: _____   WEIGHT: _____

SET 1 REPS: _____ (GOAL: 10-15) WEIGHT: _____

SET 2 REPS: _____ (GOAL: 8-12) WEIGHT: _____

SET 3 REPS: _____ (GOAL: 6-8) WEIGHT: _____

SET 4 REPS: _____ (GOAL: 4-6) WEIGHT: _____
(OPTIONAL)

3. ROPE PULLDOWN

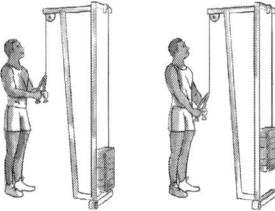

PREVIOUS BEST
(WORKOUT 47)

REPS: _____   WEIGHT: _____

SET 1 REPS: _____ (GOAL: 10-15) WEIGHT: _____

SET 2 REPS: _____ (GOAL: 8-12) WEIGHT: _____

SET 3 REPS: _____ (GOAL: 6-8) WEIGHT: _____

SET 4 REPS: _____ (GOAL: 4-6) WEIGHT: _____
(OPTIONAL)

4. DIP

(ALTERNATIVE: ASSISTED DIP
OR SEATED DIP W/ MACHINE)

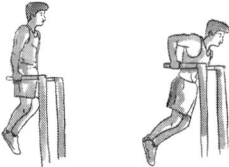

PREVIOUS BEST
(WORKOUT 41)

REPS: _____   WEIGHT: _____

SET 1 REPS: _____ (GOAL: TO FAILURE) WEIGHT: _____

SET 2 REPS: _____ (GOAL: TO FAILURE) WEIGHT: _____

SET 3 REPS: _____ (GOAL: TO FAILURE) WEIGHT: _____

SET 4 REPS: _____ (GOAL: TO FAILURE) WEIGHT: _____
(OPTIONAL)

SUPERSETS DONE TODAY (CIRCLE):
1 2 3 4

TODAY'S WORKOUT INTENSITY:
_____ / 10

Workout 54: Legs & Abs

DATE _____

1. LEG PRESS

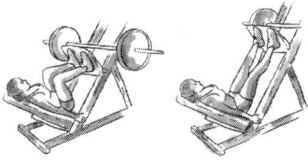

PREVIOUS BEST (WORKOUT 44) REPS: _____ WEIGHT: _____

SET 1 REPS: _____ (GOAL: 10-15) WEIGHT: _____
SET 2 REPS: _____ (GOAL: 8-12) WEIGHT: _____
SET 3 REPS: _____ (GOAL: 6-8) WEIGHT: _____
SET 4 (OPTIONAL) REPS: _____ (GOAL: 4-6) WEIGHT: _____

2. HACK SQUAT
(ALTERNATIVE: WEIGHTED LUNGE)

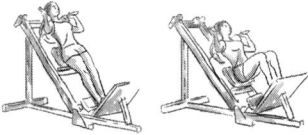

PREVIOUS BEST (WORKOUT 44) REPS: _____ WEIGHT: _____

SET 1 REPS: _____ (GOAL: 10-15) WEIGHT: _____
SET 2 REPS: _____ (GOAL: 8-12) WEIGHT: _____
SET 3 REPS: _____ (GOAL: 6-8) WEIGHT: _____
SET 4 (OPTIONAL) REPS: _____ (GOAL: 4-6) WEIGHT: _____

3. QUAD EXTENSION

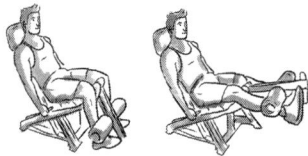

PREVIOUS BEST (WORKOUT 49) REPS: _____ WEIGHT: _____

SET 1 REPS: _____ (GOAL: 10-15) WEIGHT: _____
SET 2 REPS: _____ (GOAL: 8-12) WEIGHT: _____
SET 3 REPS: _____ (GOAL: 6-8) WEIGHT: _____
SET 4 (OPTIONAL) REPS: _____ (GOAL: 4-6) WEIGHT: _____

4. HAMSTRING EXTENSION

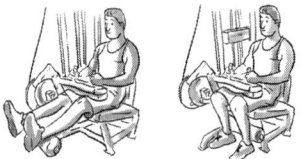

PREVIOUS BEST (WORKOUT 49) REPS: _____ WEIGHT: _____

SET 1 REPS: _____ (GOAL: 10-15) WEIGHT: _____
SET 2 REPS: _____ (GOAL: 8-12) WEIGHT: _____
SET 3 REPS: _____ (GOAL: 6-8) WEIGHT: _____
SET 4 (OPTIONAL) REPS: _____ (GOAL: 4-6) WEIGHT: _____

AMOUNT OF CARDIO DONE TODAY: _____

Workout 54: Legs & Abs

5. CALF RAISE

(ALTERNATIVE: SEATED CALF PRESS MACHINE)

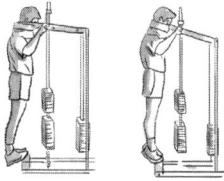

PREVIOUS BEST (WORKOUT 49)	REPS: _____		WEIGHT: _____
SET 1	REPS: _____	(GOAL: 10-15)	WEIGHT: _____
SET 2	REPS: _____	(GOAL: 8-12)	WEIGHT: _____
SET 3	REPS: _____	(GOAL: 6-8)	WEIGHT: _____
SET 4 (OPTIONAL)	REPS: _____	(GOAL: 4-6)	WEIGHT: _____

1. KNEELING CABLE CRUNCH

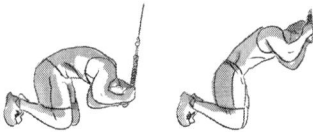

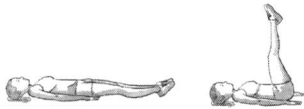

PREVIOUS BEST (WORKOUT 51)	REPS: _____		WEIGHT: _____
SET 1	REPS: _____	(GOAL: 10-20)	WEIGHT: _____
SET 2	REPS: _____	(GOAL: 10-20)	WEIGHT: _____
SET 3	REPS: _____	(GOAL: 10-20)	WEIGHT: _____

2. LEG LIFT

PREVIOUS BEST (WORKOUT 49)	REPS: _____	
SET 1	REPS: _____	(GOAL: 10-20)
SET 2	REPS: _____	(GOAL: 10-20)
SET 3	REPS: _____	(GOAL: 10-20)

3. STARFISH CRUNCH

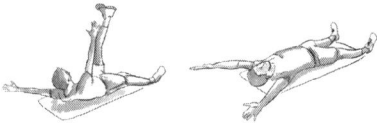

PREVIOUS BEST (WORKOUT 49)	REPS: _____	
SET 1	REPS: _____	(GOAL: 10-20 EACH SIDE)
SET 2	REPS: _____	(GOAL: 10-20 EACH SIDE)
SET 3	REPS: _____	(GOAL: 10-20 EACH SIDE)

4. PLANK

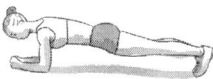

PREVIOUS BEST (WORKOUT 51)	TIME: _____	
SET 1	TIME: _____	(GOAL: 45-90 SECONDS)
SET 2	TIME: _____	(GOAL: 45-90 SECONDS)
SET 3	TIME: _____	(GOAL: 45-90 SECONDS)

SUPERSETS DONE TODAY (CIRCLE):

1   2   3   4

TODAY'S WORKOUT INTENSITY:

_____ / 10

Workout 55: Full Body Circuit

*Rest for **15-20 seconds** between each exercise, then rest for **1-2 minutes** after completing the entire circuit. Complete the full circuit **a total of 4-5 times**.*

1. JUMP

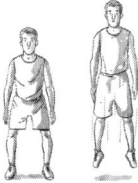

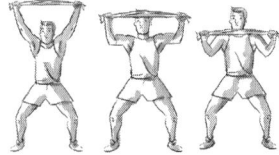

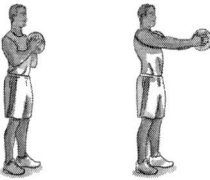

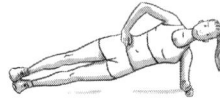

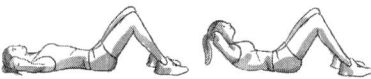

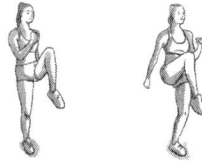

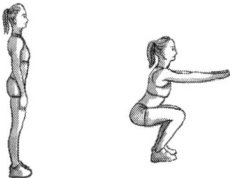

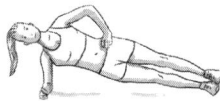

(Duration: 30 Seconds)

2. TOWEL PULL

(Duration: 30 Seconds)

3. PRAYER

(Duration: 30 Seconds)

4. SIDE PLANK

(Duration: 30 Seconds)

5. CRUNCH

(Duration: 30 Seconds)

6. HIGH KNEE

(Duration: 30 Seconds)

7. AIR SQUAT

(Duration: 30 Seconds)

8. SIDE PLANK

(Duration: 30 Seconds)

TODAY'S WORKOUT INTENSITY:

_____ / 10

<u>Pro-Tip</u>

Increase your cardio if your body fat is high.

For people trying to lose body fat - if you're at a caloric deficit, working out consistently, and still having trouble, it may be time to up your cardio.

Start by doing 20 minutes for two days a week and see how much of a difference it makes over a 1-2 week period.

If you're still not seeing visible results, up the cardio amount by one day a week, up to 6 days a week for 20 minutes each. This amount would be in addition to the weightlifting routine listed in this journal.

If you'd like some variety from the 'bodyweight' days listed in the journal, which are meant to simulate a cardio program through circuit training, you can switch to running outside or using a cardio machine (elliptical, treadmill, stairmaster, rowing machine, etc.).

You can follow a HIIT (high intensity interval training) program for any machine you choose, which shifts away from long, static cardio to bursts of intensity with recovery periods in between.

For example, one HIIT structure you could use is 30 seconds *intense*, 45 seconds *recovery*, and repeat for 20 minutes (16 cycles).

<u>Workout 56:</u> **Back** & Abs

DATE _____

1. ASSISTED PULL-UP
(ALTERNATIVE: PULL-UP OR TOWEL PULL)

PREVIOUS BEST (WORKOUT 51)   REPS: _____   WEIGHT: _____

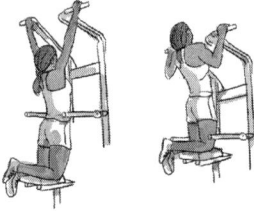

SET 1	REPS: _____	(GOAL: 10-15)	WEIGHT: _____
SET 2	REPS: _____	(GOAL: 8-12)	WEIGHT: _____
SET 3	REPS: _____	(GOAL: 6-8)	WEIGHT: _____
SET 4 (OPTIONAL)	REPS: _____	(GOAL: 4-6)	WEIGHT: _____

2. T-BAR ROW
(ALTERNATIVE: UPPER BACK ROPE PULL)

PREVIOUS BEST (WORKOUT 51)   REPS: _____   WEIGHT: _____

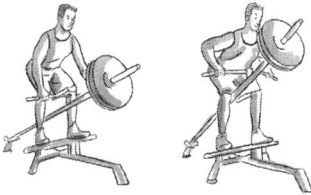

SET 1	REPS: _____	(GOAL: 10-15)	WEIGHT: _____
SET 2	REPS: _____	(GOAL: 8-12)	WEIGHT: _____
SET 3	REPS: _____	(GOAL: 6-8)	WEIGHT: _____
SET 4 (OPTIONAL)	REPS: _____	(GOAL: 4-6)	WEIGHT: _____

3. LAT PULLDOWN

PREVIOUS BEST (WORKOUT 51)   REPS: _____   WEIGHT: _____

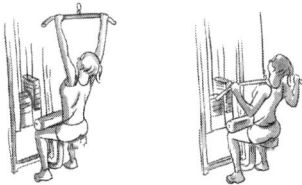

SET 1	REPS: _____	(GOAL: 10-15)	WEIGHT: _____
SET 2	REPS: _____	(GOAL: 8-12)	WEIGHT: _____
SET 3	REPS: _____	(GOAL: 6-8)	WEIGHT: _____
SET 4 (OPTIONAL)	REPS: _____	(GOAL: 4-6)	WEIGHT: _____

4. CLOSE GRIP CABLE ROW
(ALTERNATIVE: PULL-UP OR LAT ROW)

PREVIOUS BEST (WORKOUT 51)   REPS: _____   WEIGHT: _____

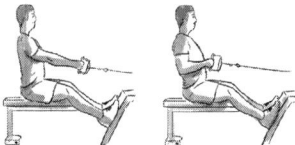

SET 1	REPS: _____	(GOAL: 10-15)	WEIGHT: _____
SET 2	REPS: _____	(GOAL: 8-12)	WEIGHT: _____
SET 3	REPS: _____	(GOAL: 6-8)	WEIGHT: _____
SET 4 (OPTIONAL)	REPS: _____	(GOAL: 4-6)	WEIGHT: _____

AMOUNT OF CARDIO DONE TODAY:
_____

Workout 56: Back & Abs

5. UPPER BACK ROPE PULL

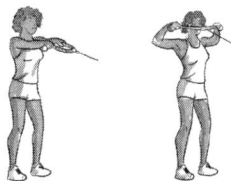

PREVIOUS BEST (WORKOUT 51) REPS: _____   WEIGHT: _____

SET 1	REPS: _____	(GOAL: 10-15)	WEIGHT: _____
SET 2	REPS: _____	(GOAL: 8-12)	WEIGHT: _____
SET 3	REPS: _____	(GOAL: 6-8)	WEIGHT: _____
SET 4 (OPTIONAL)	REPS: _____	(GOAL: 4-6)	WEIGHT: _____

1. KNEELING CABLE CRUNCH

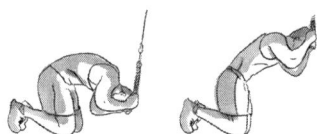

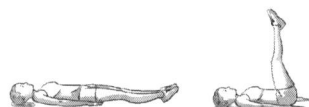

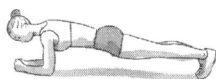

PREVIOUS BEST (WORKOUT 54) REPS: _____   WEIGHT: _____

SET 1	REPS: _____	(GOAL: 10-20)	WEIGHT: _____
SET 2	REPS: _____	(GOAL: 10-20)	WEIGHT: _____
SET 3	REPS: _____	(GOAL: 10-20)	WEIGHT: _____

2. LEG LIFT

PREVIOUS BEST (WORKOUT 54) REPS: _____

SET 1	REPS: _____	(GOAL: 10-20)
SET 2	REPS: _____	(GOAL: 10-20)
SET 3	REPS: _____	(GOAL: 10-20)

3. STARFISH CRUNCH

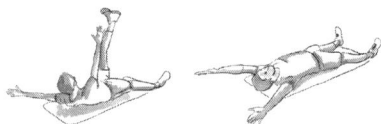

PREVIOUS BEST (WORKOUT 54) REPS: _____

SET 1	REPS: _____	(GOAL: 10-20 EACH SIDE)
SET 2	REPS: _____	(GOAL: 10-20 EACH SIDE)
SET 3	REPS: _____	(GOAL: 10-20 EACH SIDE)

4. PLANK

PREVIOUS BEST (WORKOUT 54) TIME: _____

SET 1	TIME: _____	(GOAL: 45-90 SECONDS)
SET 2	TIME: _____	(GOAL: 45-90 SECONDS)
SET 3	TIME: _____	(GOAL: 45-90 SECONDS)

SUPERSETS DONE TODAY (CIRCLE):
1   2   3   4

TODAY'S WORKOUT INTENSITY:
_____ / 10

Workout 57: Chest & Biceps

DATE _____

1. FLAT BENCH PRESS

(ALTERNATIVE: FLAT BENCH DUMBBELL PRESS)

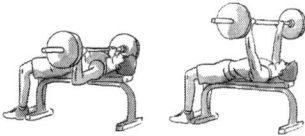

PREVIOUS BEST (WORKOUT 52) REPS: _____   WEIGHT: _____

SET 1 REPS: _____ (GOAL: 10-15)   WEIGHT: _____
SET 2 REPS: _____ (GOAL: 8-12)   WEIGHT: _____
SET 3 REPS: _____ (GOAL: 6-8)   WEIGHT: _____
SET 4 (OPTIONAL) REPS: _____ (GOAL: 4-6)   WEIGHT: _____

2. DECLINE BENCH PRESS

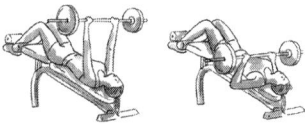

PREVIOUS BEST (WORKOUT 37) REPS: _____   WEIGHT: _____

SET 1 REPS: _____ (GOAL: 10-15)   WEIGHT: _____
SET 2 REPS: _____ (GOAL: 8-12)   WEIGHT: _____
SET 3 REPS: _____ (GOAL: 6-8)   WEIGHT: _____
SET 4 (OPTIONAL) REPS: _____ (GOAL: 4-6)   WEIGHT: _____

3. INCLINE BENCH PRESS

(ALTERNATIVE: INCLINE BENCH PRESS)

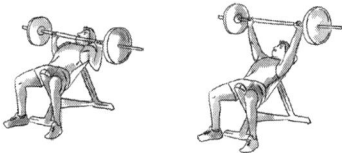

PREVIOUS BEST (WORKOUT 52) REPS: _____   WEIGHT: _____

SET 1 REPS: _____ (GOAL: 10-15)   WEIGHT: _____
SET 2 REPS: _____ (GOAL: 8-12)   WEIGHT: _____
SET 3 REPS: _____ (GOAL: 6-8)   WEIGHT: _____
SET 4 (OPTIONAL) REPS: _____ (GOAL: 4-6)   WEIGHT: _____

4. FLAT BENCH DUMBBELL FLY

(ALTERNATIVE: CHEST FLY W/ MACHINE)

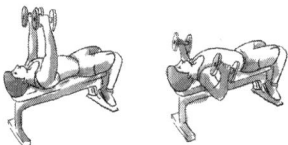

PREVIOUS BEST (WORKOUT 52) REPS: _____   WEIGHT: _____

SET 1 REPS: _____ (GOAL: 10-15)   WEIGHT: _____
SET 2 REPS: _____ (GOAL: 8-12)   WEIGHT: _____
SET 3 REPS: _____ (GOAL: 6-8)   WEIGHT: _____
SET 4 (OPTIONAL) REPS: _____ (GOAL: 4-6)   WEIGHT: _____

AMOUNT OF CARDIO DONE TODAY: _____

<u>Workout 57:</u> Chest & **Biceps**

1. PREACHER CURL

(ALTERNATIVE: SEATED DUMBBELL CURL)

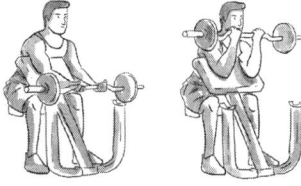

PREVIOUS BEST
(WORKOUT 52)

REPS: _____ WEIGHT: _____

SET 1 REPS: _____ (GOAL: 10-15) WEIGHT: _____

SET 2 REPS: _____ (GOAL: 8-12) WEIGHT: _____

SET 3 REPS: _____ (GOAL: 6-8) WEIGHT: _____

SET 4 REPS: _____ (GOAL: 4-6) WEIGHT: _____
[OPTIONAL]

2. DUMBBELL HAMMER CURL

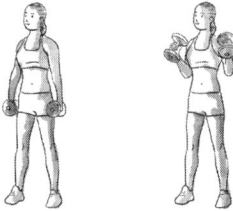

PREVIOUS BEST
(WORKOUT 46)

REPS: _____ WEIGHT: _____

SET 1 REPS: _____ (GOAL: 10-15) WEIGHT: _____

SET 2 REPS: _____ (GOAL: 8-12) WEIGHT: _____

SET 3 REPS: _____ (GOAL: 6-8) WEIGHT: _____

SET 4 REPS: _____ (GOAL: 4-6) WEIGHT: _____
[OPTIONAL]

3. CONCENTRATION CURL

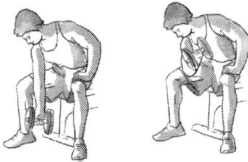

PREVIOUS BEST
(WORKOUT 46)

REPS: _____ WEIGHT: _____

SET 1 REPS: _____ (GOAL: 10-15) WEIGHT: _____

SET 2 REPS: _____ (GOAL: 8-12) WEIGHT: _____

SET 3 REPS: _____ (GOAL: 6-8) WEIGHT: _____

SET 4 REPS: _____ (GOAL: 4-6) WEIGHT: _____
[OPTIONAL]

4. OVERHEAD CABLE CURL

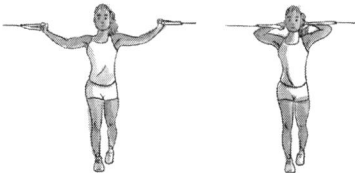

PREVIOUS BEST
(WORKOUT 52)

REPS: _____ WEIGHT: _____

SET 1 REPS: _____ (GOAL: 10-15) WEIGHT: _____

SET 2 REPS: _____ (GOAL: 8-12) WEIGHT: _____

SET 3 REPS: _____ (GOAL: 6-8) WEIGHT: _____

SET 4 REPS: _____ (GOAL: 4-6) WEIGHT: _____
[OPTIONAL]

SUPERSETS DONE TODAY (CIRCLE):

1   2   3   4

TODAY'S WORKOUT INTENSITY:

_____ / 10

Workout 58: Shoulders & Triceps

DATE _____

1. LATERAL DUMBBELL RAISE

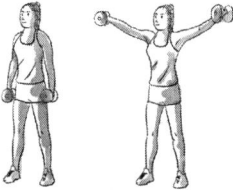

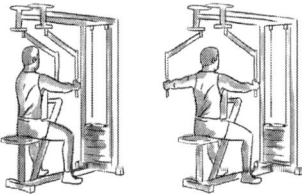

PREVIOUS BEST (WORKOUT 53)   REPS: _____   WEIGHT: _____

SET 1   REPS: _____ (GOAL: 10-15)   WEIGHT: _____

SET 2   REPS: _____ (GOAL: 8-12)   WEIGHT: _____

SET 3   REPS: _____ (GOAL: 6-8)   WEIGHT: _____

SET 4 (OPTIONAL)   REPS: _____ (GOAL: 4-6)   WEIGHT: _____

2. FRONT DUMBBELL RAISE

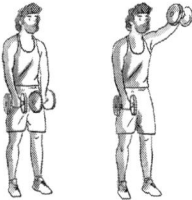

PREVIOUS BEST (WORKOUT 53)   REPS: _____   WEIGHT: _____

SET 1   REPS: _____ (GOAL: 10-15)   WEIGHT: _____

SET 2   REPS: _____ (GOAL: 8-12)   WEIGHT: _____

SET 3   REPS: _____ (GOAL: 6-8)   WEIGHT: _____

SET 4 (OPTIONAL)   REPS: _____ (GOAL: 4-6)   WEIGHT: _____

3. REVERSE FLY

PREVIOUS BEST (WORKOUT 53)   REPS: _____   WEIGHT: _____

SET 1   REPS: _____ (GOAL: 10-15)   WEIGHT: _____

SET 2   REPS: _____ (GOAL: 8-12)   WEIGHT: _____

SET 3   REPS: _____ (GOAL: 6-8)   WEIGHT: _____

SET 4 (OPTIONAL)   REPS: _____ (GOAL: 4-6)   WEIGHT: _____

4. SEATED DUMBBELL PRESS

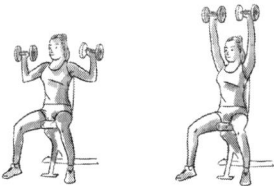

PREVIOUS BEST (WORKOUT 53)   REPS: _____   WEIGHT: _____

SET 1   REPS: _____ (GOAL: 10-15)   WEIGHT: _____

SET 2   REPS: _____ (GOAL: 8-12)   WEIGHT: _____

SET 3   REPS: _____ (GOAL: 6-8)   WEIGHT: _____

SET 4 (OPTIONAL)   REPS: _____ (GOAL: 4-6)   WEIGHT: _____

AMOUNT OF CARDIO DONE TODAY: _____

Workout 58: Shoulders & Triceps

1. SKULL CRUSHER

(ALTERNATIVE: CLOSE GRIP BENCH PRESS OR DUMBBELL PULLOVER)

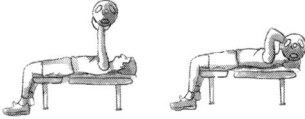

PREVIOUS BEST (WORKOUT 53)

REPS: _____ WEIGHT: _____

SET 1 REPS: _____ (GOAL: 10-15) WEIGHT: _____

SET 2 REPS: _____ (GOAL: 8-12) WEIGHT: _____

SET 3 REPS: _____ (GOAL: 6-8) WEIGHT: _____

SET 4 (OPTIONAL) REPS: _____ (GOAL: 4-6) WEIGHT: _____

2. OVERHEAD DUMBBELL EXTENSION

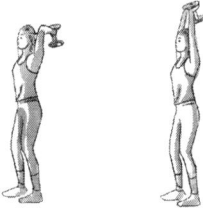

PREVIOUS BEST (WORKOUT 53)

REPS: _____ WEIGHT: _____

SET 1 REPS: _____ (GOAL: 10-15) WEIGHT: _____

SET 2 REPS: _____ (GOAL: 8-12) WEIGHT: _____

SET 3 REPS: _____ (GOAL: 6-8) WEIGHT: _____

SET 4 (OPTIONAL) REPS: _____ (GOAL: 4-6) WEIGHT: _____

3. ROPE PULLDOWN

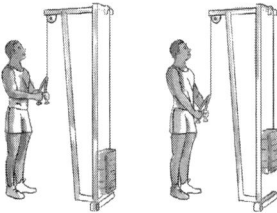

PREVIOUS BEST (WORKOUT 53)

REPS: _____ WEIGHT: _____

SET 1 REPS: _____ (GOAL: 10-15) WEIGHT: _____

SET 2 REPS: _____ (GOAL: 8-12) WEIGHT: _____

SET 3 REPS: _____ (GOAL: 6-8) WEIGHT: _____

SET 4 (OPTIONAL) REPS: _____ (GOAL: 4-6) WEIGHT: _____

4. DIP

(ALTERNATIVE: ASSISTED DIP OR SEATED DIP W/ MACHINE)

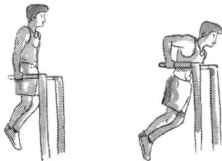

PREVIOUS BEST (WORKOUT 53)

REPS: _____ WEIGHT: _____

SET 1 REPS: _____ (GOAL: TO FAILURE) WEIGHT: _____

SET 2 REPS: _____ (GOAL: TO FAILURE) WEIGHT: _____

SET 3 REPS: _____ (GOAL: TO FAILURE) WEIGHT: _____

SET 4 (OPTIONAL) REPS: _____ (GOAL: TO FAILURE) WEIGHT: _____

SUPERSETS DONE TODAY (CIRCLE):

1 2 3 4

TODAY'S WORKOUT INTENSITY:

_____ / 10

Workout 59: Legs & Abs

DATE _____

1. DEADLIFT

(ALTERNATIVE: LEG PRESS)

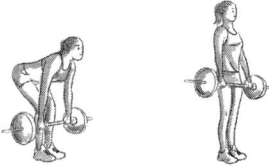

PREVIOUS BEST (WORKOUT 49)   REPS: _____   WEIGHT: _____

SET 1	REPS: _____	(GOAL: 10-15)	WEIGHT: _____
SET 2	REPS: _____	(GOAL: 8-12)	WEIGHT: _____
SET 3	REPS: _____	(GOAL: 6-8)	WEIGHT: _____
SET 4 (OPTIONAL)	REPS: _____	(GOAL: 4-6)	WEIGHT: _____

2. BARBELL SQUAT

(ALTERNATIVE: HACK SQUAT)

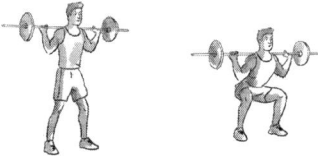

PREVIOUS BEST (WORKOUT 49)   REPS: _____   WEIGHT: _____

SET 1	REPS: _____	(GOAL: 10-15)	WEIGHT: _____
SET 2	REPS: _____	(GOAL: 8-12)	WEIGHT: _____
SET 3	REPS: _____	(GOAL: 6-8)	WEIGHT: _____
SET 4 (OPTIONAL)	REPS: _____	(GOAL: 4-6)	WEIGHT: _____

3. WEIGHTED LUNGE

(ALTERNATIVE: QUAD EXTENSION)

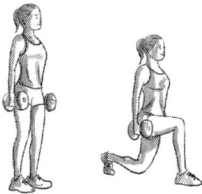

PREVIOUS BEST (WORKOUT 44)   REPS: _____   WEIGHT: _____

SET 1	REPS: _____	(GOAL: 10-15)	WEIGHT: _____
SET 2	REPS: _____	(GOAL: 8-12)	WEIGHT: _____
SET 3	REPS: _____	(GOAL: 6-8)	WEIGHT: _____
SET 4 (OPTIONAL)	REPS: _____	(GOAL: 4-6)	WEIGHT: _____

4. HAMSTRING EXTENSION

PREVIOUS BEST (WORKOUT 54)   REPS: _____   WEIGHT: _____

SET 1	REPS: _____	(GOAL: 10-15)	WEIGHT: _____
SET 2	REPS: _____	(GOAL: 8-12)	WEIGHT: _____
SET 3	REPS: _____	(GOAL: 6-8)	WEIGHT: _____
SET 4 (OPTIONAL)	REPS: _____	(GOAL: 4-6)	WEIGHT: _____

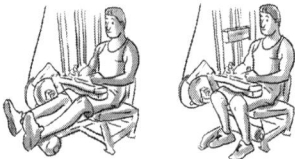

AMOUNT OF CARDIO DONE TODAY: _____

190

Workout 59: Legs & Abs

5. CALF RAISE

(ALTERNATIVE: SEATED CALF PRESS MACHINE)

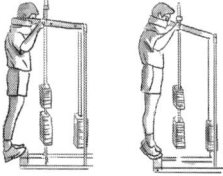

PREVIOUS BEST (WORKOUT 54)

REPS: _____   WEIGHT: _____

SET 1	REPS: _____	(GOAL: 10-15)	WEIGHT: _____
SET 2	REPS: _____	(GOAL: 8-12)	WEIGHT: _____
SET 3	REPS: _____	(GOAL: 6-8)	WEIGHT: _____
SET 4 (OPTIONAL)	REPS: _____	(GOAL: 4-6)	WEIGHT: _____

1. KNEELING CABLE CRUNCH

PREVIOUS BEST (WORKOUT 56)

REPS: _____   WEIGHT: _____

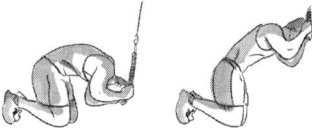

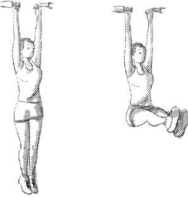

SET 1	REPS: _____	(GOAL: 10-20)	WEIGHT: _____
SET 2	REPS: _____	(GOAL: 10-20)	WEIGHT: _____
SET 3	REPS: _____	(GOAL: 10-20)	WEIGHT: _____

2. HANGING LEG LIFT

PREVIOUS BEST (WORKOUT 51)

REPS: _____

SET 1	REPS: _____	(GOAL: 10-20)
SET 2	REPS: _____	(GOAL: 10-20)
SET 3	REPS: _____	(GOAL: 10-20)

3. RUSSIAN TWIST

PREVIOUS BEST (WORKOUT 44)

REPS: _____

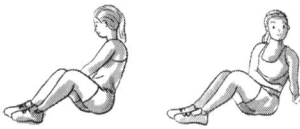

SET 1	REPS: _____	(GOAL: 10-20 EACH SIDE)
SET 2	REPS: _____	(GOAL: 10-20 EACH SIDE)
SET 3	REPS: _____	(GOAL: 10-20 EACH SIDE)

4. PLANK

PREVIOUS BEST (WORKOUT 56)

TIME: _____

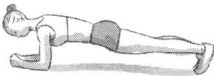

SET 1	TIME: _____	(GOAL: 45-90 SECONDS)
SET 2	TIME: _____	(GOAL: 45-90 SECONDS)
SET 3	TIME: _____	(GOAL: 45-90 SECONDS)

SUPERSETS DONE TODAY (CIRCLE):

1   2   3   4

TODAY'S WORKOUT INTENSITY:

_____ / 10

Workout 60: Full Body Circuit

Rest for 15-20 seconds between each exercise, then rest for 1-2 minutes after completing the entire circuit. Complete the full circuit a total of 4-5 times.

1. RUN IN PLACE

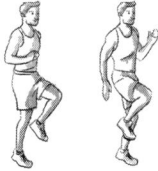

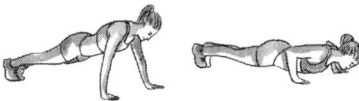

(Duration: 30 Seconds)

2. MOUNTAIN CLIMBER

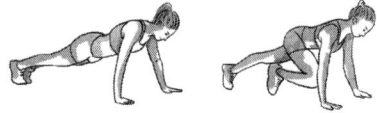

(Duration: 30 Seconds)

3. STARFISH CRUNCH

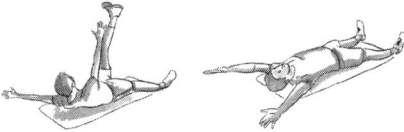

(Duration: 30 Seconds)

4. BICYCLE CRUNCH

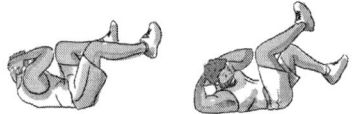

(Duration: 30 Seconds)

5. ALTERNATING LUNGE

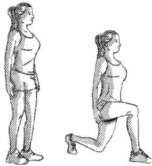

(Duration: 30 Seconds)

6. TOWEL SNATCH

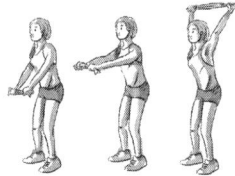

(Duration: 30 Seconds)

7. PUSH-UP

(Duration: 30 Seconds)

8. VERTICAL LEAP

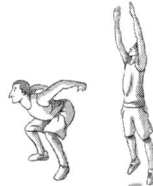

(Duration: 30 Seconds)

TODAY'S WORKOUT INTENSITY:

_____ / 10

<u>Check-In</u> ⊘

How do I feel about the way I look now compared to when I started?

_____

_____

_____

_____

Which body parts am I happier with?

_____

_____

_____

_____

Which body parts do I need to work more (maybe a bonus day for those muscles)?

_____

_____

_____

_____

Am I noticing any changes in my mental attitude in general (happier, more confident, etc.)?

_____

_____

_____

_____

EXERCISE
GUIDE

https://HabitNest.link/lifting61

Workout 61: Back & Abs

DATE _____

1. ASSISTED PULL-UP
(ALTERNATIVE: PULL-UP OR TOWEL PULL)

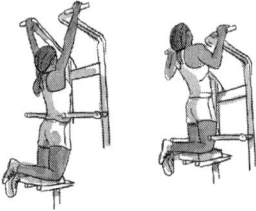

PREVIOUS BEST
(WORKOUT 56)   REPS: _____   WEIGHT: _____

SET 1   REPS: _____   (GOAL: 10-15)   WEIGHT: _____
SET 2   REPS: _____   (GOAL: 8-12)   WEIGHT: _____
SET 3   REPS: _____   (GOAL: 6-8)   WEIGHT: _____
SET 4   REPS: _____   (GOAL: 4-6)   WEIGHT: _____
(OPTIONAL)

2. T-BAR ROW
(ALTERNATIVE: UPPER BACK ROPE PULL)

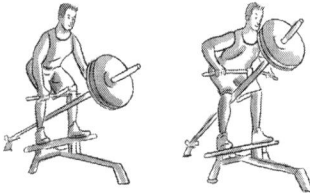

PREVIOUS BEST
(WORKOUT 56)   REPS: _____   WEIGHT: _____

SET 1   REPS: _____   (GOAL: 10-15)   WEIGHT: _____
SET 2   REPS: _____   (GOAL: 8-12)   WEIGHT: _____
SET 3   REPS: _____   (GOAL: 6-8)   WEIGHT: _____
SET 4   REPS: _____   (GOAL: 4-6)   WEIGHT: _____
(OPTIONAL)

3. LAT PULLDOWN

PREVIOUS BEST
(WORKOUT 56)   REPS: _____   WEIGHT: _____

SET 1   REPS: _____   (GOAL: 10-15)   WEIGHT: _____
SET 2   REPS: _____   (GOAL: 8-12)   WEIGHT: _____
SET 3   REPS: _____   (GOAL: 6-8)   WEIGHT: _____
SET 4   REPS: _____   (GOAL: 4-6)   WEIGHT: _____
(OPTIONAL)

4. CLOSE GRIP CABLE ROW
(ALTERNATIVE: PULL-UP OR LAT ROW)

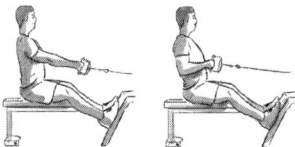

PREVIOUS BEST
(WORKOUT 56)   REPS: _____   WEIGHT: _____

SET 1   REPS: _____   (GOAL: 10-15)   WEIGHT: _____
SET 2   REPS: _____   (GOAL: 8-12)   WEIGHT: _____
SET 3   REPS: _____   (GOAL: 6-8)   WEIGHT: _____
SET 4   REPS: _____   (GOAL: 4-6)   WEIGHT: _____
(OPTIONAL)

AMOUNT OF CARDIO DONE TODAY: _____

194

Workout 61: Back & Abs

5. UPPER BACK ROPE PULL

PREVIOUS BEST (WORKOUT 56) REPS: _____   WEIGHT: _____

SET 1 REPS: _____ (GOAL: 10-15)   WEIGHT: _____

SET 2 REPS: _____ (GOAL: 8-12)   WEIGHT: _____

SET 3 REPS: _____ (GOAL: 6-8)   WEIGHT: _____

SET 4 (OPTIONAL) REPS: _____ (GOAL: 4-6)   WEIGHT: _____

1. KNEELING CABLE CRUNCH

PREVIOUS BEST (WORKOUT 59) REPS: _____   WEIGHT: _____

SET 1 REPS: _____ (GOAL: 10-20)   WEIGHT: _____

SET 2 REPS: _____ (GOAL: 10-20)   WEIGHT: _____

SET 3 REPS: _____ (GOAL: 10-20)   WEIGHT: _____

2. LEG LIFT

PREVIOUS BEST (WORKOUT 56) REPS: _____

SET 1 REPS: _____ (GOAL: 10-20)

SET 2 REPS: _____ (GOAL: 10-20)

SET 3 REPS: _____ (GOAL: 10-20)

3. STARFISH CRUNCH

PREVIOUS BEST (WORKOUT 56) REPS: _____

SET 1 REPS: _____ (GOAL: 10-20 EACH SIDE)

SET 2 REPS: _____ (GOAL: 10-20 EACH SIDE)

SET 3 REPS: _____ (GOAL: 10-20 EACH SIDE)

4. PLANK

PREVIOUS BEST (WORKOUT 59) TIME: _____

SET 1 TIME: _____ (GOAL: 45-90 SECONDS)

SET 2 TIME: _____ (GOAL: 45-90 SECONDS)

SET 3 TIME: _____ (GOAL: 45-90 SECONDS)

SUPERSETS DONE TODAY (CIRCLE):
1   2   3   4

TODAY'S WORKOUT INTENSITY:
_____ / 10

Workout 62: Chest & Biceps

DATE _____

1. FLAT BENCH PRESS

(ALTERNATIVE: FLAT BENCH DUMBBELL PRESS)

PREVIOUS BEST
(WORKOUT 57) REPS: _____   WEIGHT: _____

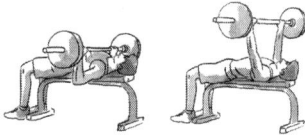

SET 1	REPS: _____	(GOAL: 10-15)	WEIGHT: _____
SET 2	REPS: _____	(GOAL: 8-12)	WEIGHT: _____
SET 3	REPS: _____	(GOAL: 6-8)	WEIGHT: _____
SET 4 (OPTIONAL)	REPS: _____	(GOAL: 4-6)	WEIGHT: _____

2. DECLINE BENCH PRESS

PREVIOUS BEST
(WORKOUT 57) REPS: _____   WEIGHT: _____

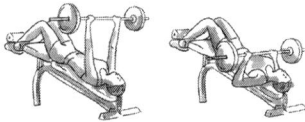

SET 1	REPS: _____	(GOAL: 10-15)	WEIGHT: _____
SET 2	REPS: _____	(GOAL: 8-12)	WEIGHT: _____
SET 3	REPS: _____	(GOAL: 6-8)	WEIGHT: _____
SET 4 (OPTIONAL)	REPS: _____	(GOAL: 4-6)	WEIGHT: _____

3. INCLINE BENCH PRESS

(ALTERNATIVE: INCLINE DUMBBELL PRESS)

PREVIOUS BEST
(WORKOUT 57) REPS: _____   WEIGHT: _____

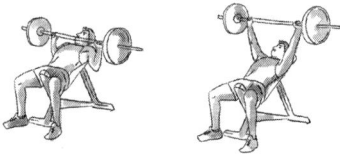

SET 1	REPS: _____	(GOAL: 10-15)	WEIGHT: _____
SET 2	REPS: _____	(GOAL: 8-12)	WEIGHT: _____
SET 3	REPS: _____	(GOAL: 6-8)	WEIGHT: _____
SET 4 (OPTIONAL)	REPS: _____	(GOAL: 4-6)	WEIGHT: _____

4. FLAT BENCH DUMBBELL FLY

(ALTERNATIVE: CHEST FLY W/ MACHINE)

PREVIOUS BEST
(WORKOUT 57) REPS: _____   WEIGHT: _____

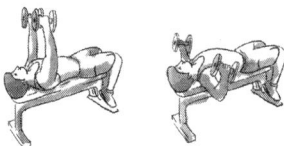

SET 1	REPS: _____	(GOAL: 10-15)	WEIGHT: _____
SET 2	REPS: _____	(GOAL: 8-12)	WEIGHT: _____
SET 3	REPS: _____	(GOAL: 6-8)	WEIGHT: _____
SET 4 (OPTIONAL)	REPS: _____	(GOAL: 4-6)	WEIGHT: _____

AMOUNT OF CARDIO DONE TODAY: _____

Workout 62: Chest & Biceps

1. PREACHER CURL

(ALTERNATIVE: SEATED DUMBBELL CURL)

PREVIOUS BEST
(WORKOUT 57)

REPS: _____   WEIGHT: _____

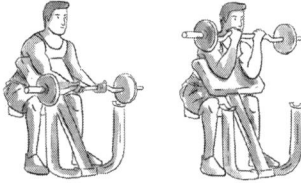

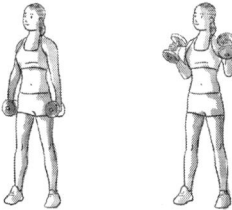

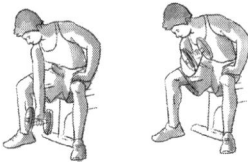

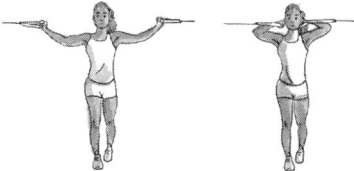

SET 1   REPS: _____ (GOAL: 10-15)   WEIGHT: _____
SET 2   REPS: _____ (GOAL: 8-12)   WEIGHT: _____
SET 3   REPS: _____ (GOAL: 6-8)   WEIGHT: _____
SET 4   REPS: _____ (GOAL: 4-6)   WEIGHT: _____
(OPTIONAL)

2. DUMBBELL HAMMER CURL

PREVIOUS BEST
(WORKOUT 57)

REPS: _____   WEIGHT: _____

SET 1   REPS: _____ (GOAL: 10-15)   WEIGHT: _____
SET 2   REPS: _____ (GOAL: 8-12)   WEIGHT: _____
SET 3   REPS: _____ (GOAL: 6-8)   WEIGHT: _____
SET 4   REPS: _____ (GOAL: 4-6)   WEIGHT: _____
(OPTIONAL)

3. CONCENTRATION CURL

PREVIOUS BEST
(WORKOUT 57)

REPS: _____   WEIGHT: _____

SET 1   REPS: _____ (GOAL: 10-15)   WEIGHT: _____
SET 2   REPS: _____ (GOAL: 8-12)   WEIGHT: _____
SET 3   REPS: _____ (GOAL: 6-8)   WEIGHT: _____
SET 4   REPS: _____ (GOAL: 4-6)   WEIGHT: _____
(OPTIONAL)

4. OVERHEAD CABLE CURL

PREVIOUS BEST
(WORKOUT 57)

REPS: _____   WEIGHT: _____

SET 1   REPS: _____ (GOAL: 10-15)   WEIGHT: _____
SET 2   REPS: _____ (GOAL: 8-12)   WEIGHT: _____
SET 3   REPS: _____ (GOAL: 6-8)   WEIGHT: _____
SET 4   REPS: _____ (GOAL: 4-6)   WEIGHT: _____
(OPTIONAL)

SUPERSETS DONE TODAY (CIRCLE):

1   2   3   4

TODAY'S WORKOUT INTENSITY:

_____ / 10

EXERCISE
GUIDE

https://HabitNest.link/lifting63

Workout 63: Shoulders & Triceps

DATE _____

1. LATERAL DUMBBELL RAISE

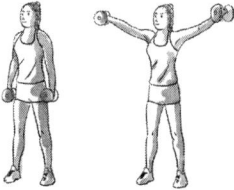

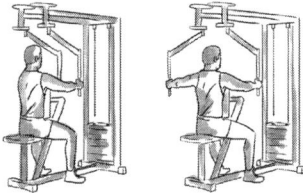

PREVIOUS BEST (WORKOUT 58)   REPS: _____   WEIGHT: _____

SET 1   REPS: _____ (GOAL: 10-15)   WEIGHT: _____

SET 2   REPS: _____ (GOAL: 8-12)   WEIGHT: _____

SET 3   REPS: _____ (GOAL: 6-8)   WEIGHT: _____

SET 4 (OPTIONAL)   REPS: _____ (GOAL: 4-6)   WEIGHT: _____

2. FRONT DUMBBELL RAISE

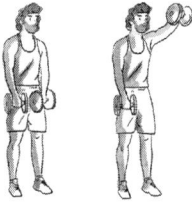

PREVIOUS BEST (WORKOUT 58)   REPS: _____   WEIGHT: _____

SET 1   REPS: _____ (GOAL: 10-15)   WEIGHT: _____

SET 2   REPS: _____ (GOAL: 8-12)   WEIGHT: _____

SET 3   REPS: _____ (GOAL: 6-8)   WEIGHT: _____

SET 4 (OPTIONAL)   REPS: _____ (GOAL: 4-6)   WEIGHT: _____

3. REVERSE FLY

PREVIOUS BEST (WORKOUT 58)   REPS: _____   WEIGHT: _____

SET 1   REPS: _____ (GOAL: 10-15)   WEIGHT: _____

SET 2   REPS: _____ (GOAL: 8-12)   WEIGHT: _____

SET 3   REPS: _____ (GOAL: 6-8)   WEIGHT: _____

SET 4 (OPTIONAL)   REPS: _____ (GOAL: 4-6)   WEIGHT: _____

4. SEATED DUMBBELL PRESS

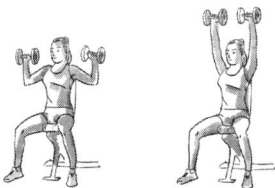

PREVIOUS BEST (WORKOUT 58)   REPS: _____   WEIGHT: _____

SET 1   REPS: _____ (GOAL: 10-15)   WEIGHT: _____

SET 2   REPS: _____ (GOAL: 8-12)   WEIGHT: _____

SET 3   REPS: _____ (GOAL: 6-8)   WEIGHT: _____

SET 4 (OPTIONAL)   REPS: _____ (GOAL: 4-6)   WEIGHT: _____

AMOUNT OF CARDIO DONE TODAY: _____

Workout 63: Shoulders & Triceps

1. SKULL CRUSHER

(ALTERNATIVE: CLOSE GRIP BENCH PRESS OR DUMBBELL PULLOVER)

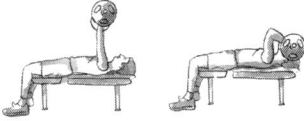

PREVIOUS BEST (WORKOUT 58)

REPS: _____ WEIGHT: _____

SET 1 REPS: _____ (GOAL: 10-15) WEIGHT: _____

SET 2 REPS: _____ (GOAL: 8-12) WEIGHT: _____

SET 3 REPS: _____ (GOAL: 6-8) WEIGHT: _____

SET 4 REPS: _____ (GOAL: 4-6) WEIGHT: _____
[OPTIONAL]

2. OVERHEAD DUMBBELL EXTENSION

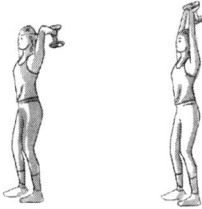

PREVIOUS BEST (WORKOUT 58)

REPS: _____ WEIGHT: _____

SET 1 REPS: _____ (GOAL: 10-15) WEIGHT: _____

SET 2 REPS: _____ (GOAL: 8-12) WEIGHT: _____

SET 3 REPS: _____ (GOAL: 6-8) WEIGHT: _____

SET 4 REPS: _____ (GOAL: 4-6) WEIGHT: _____
[OPTIONAL]

3. ROPE PULLDOWN

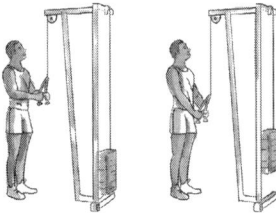

PREVIOUS BEST (WORKOUT 58)

REPS: _____ WEIGHT: _____

SET 1 REPS: _____ (GOAL: 10-15) WEIGHT: _____

SET 2 REPS: _____ (GOAL: 8-12) WEIGHT: _____

SET 3 REPS: _____ (GOAL: 6-8) WEIGHT: _____

SET 4 REPS: _____ (GOAL: 4-6) WEIGHT: _____
[OPTIONAL]

4. DIP

(ALTERNATIVE: ASSISTED DIP OR SEATED DIP W/ MACHINE)

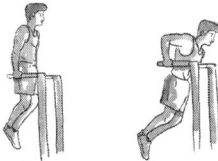

PREVIOUS BEST (WORKOUT 58)

REPS: _____ WEIGHT: _____

SET 1 REPS: _____ (GOAL: TO FAILURE) WEIGHT: _____

SET 2 REPS: _____ (GOAL: TO FAILURE) WEIGHT: _____

SET 3 REPS: _____ (GOAL: TO FAILURE) WEIGHT: _____

SET 4 REPS: _____ (GOAL: TO FAILURE) WEIGHT: _____
[OPTIONAL]

SUPERSETS DONE TODAY (CIRCLE):

1   2   3   4

TODAY'S WORKOUT INTENSITY:

_____ / 10

Workout 64: Legs & Abs

DATE _____

1. DEADLIFT

(ALTERNATIVE: LEG PRESS)

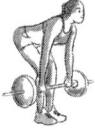

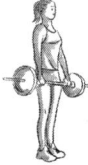

PREVIOUS BEST
(WORKOUT 59)

REPS: _____   WEIGHT: _____

SET 1   REPS: _____   (GOAL: 10-15)   WEIGHT: _____

SET 2   REPS: _____   (GOAL: 8-12)   WEIGHT: _____

SET 3   REPS: _____   (GOAL: 6-8)   WEIGHT: _____

SET 4   REPS: _____   (GOAL: 4-6)   WEIGHT: _____
(OPTIONAL)

2. BARBELL SQUAT

(ALTERNATIVE: HACK SQUAT)

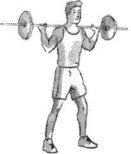

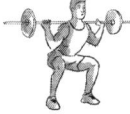

PREVIOUS BEST
(WORKOUT 59)

REPS: _____   WEIGHT: _____

SET 1   REPS: _____   (GOAL: 10-15)   WEIGHT: _____

SET 2   REPS: _____   (GOAL: 8-12)   WEIGHT: _____

SET 3   REPS: _____   (GOAL: 6-8)   WEIGHT: _____

SET 4   REPS: _____   (GOAL: 4-6)   WEIGHT: _____
(OPTIONAL)

3. WEIGHTED LUNGE

(ALTERNATIVE: QUAD EXTENSION)

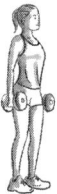

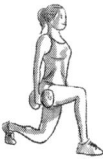

PREVIOUS BEST
(WORKOUT 59)

REPS: _____   WEIGHT: _____

SET 1   REPS: _____   (GOAL: 10-15)   WEIGHT: _____

SET 2   REPS: _____   (GOAL: 8-12)   WEIGHT: _____

SET 3   REPS: _____   (GOAL: 6-8)   WEIGHT: _____

SET 4   REPS: _____   (GOAL: 4-6)   WEIGHT: _____
(OPTIONAL)

4. HAMSTRING EXTENSION

PREVIOUS BEST
(WORKOUT 59)

REPS: _____   WEIGHT: _____

SET 1   REPS: _____   (GOAL: 10-15)   WEIGHT: _____

SET 2   REPS: _____   (GOAL: 8-12)   WEIGHT: _____

SET 3   REPS: _____   (GOAL: 6-8)   WEIGHT: _____

SET 4   REPS: _____   (GOAL: 4-6)   WEIGHT: _____
(OPTIONAL)

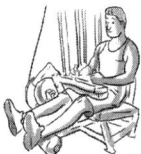

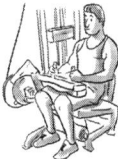

AMOUNT OF CARDIO DONE TODAY:
_____

Workout 64: Legs & Abs

5. CALF RAISE

(ALTERNATIVE: SEATED CALF PRESS MACHINE)

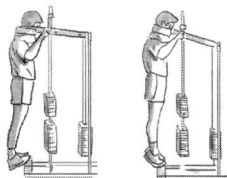

PREVIOUS BEST (WORKOUT 59)	REPS: _____		WEIGHT: _____	
SET 1	REPS: _____	(GOAL: 10-15)	WEIGHT: _____	
SET 2	REPS: _____	(GOAL: 8-12)	WEIGHT: _____	
SET 3	REPS: _____	(GOAL: 6-8)	WEIGHT: _____	
SET 4 (OPTIONAL)	REPS: _____	(GOAL: 4-6)	WEIGHT: _____	

1. KNEELING CABLE CRUNCH

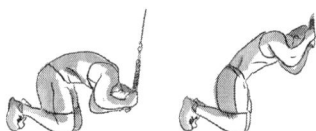

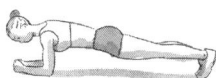

PREVIOUS BEST (WORKOUT 61)	REPS: _____		WEIGHT: _____	
SET 1	REPS: _____	(GOAL: 10-20)	WEIGHT: _____	
SET 2	REPS: _____	(GOAL: 10-20)	WEIGHT: _____	
SET 3	REPS: _____	(GOAL: 10-20)	WEIGHT: _____	

2. HANGING LEG LIFT

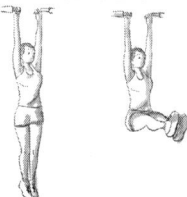

PREVIOUS BEST (WORKOUT 59)	REPS: _____	
SET 1	REPS: _____	(GOAL: 10-20)
SET 2	REPS: _____	(GOAL: 10-20)
SET 3	REPS: _____	(GOAL: 10-20)

3. RUSSIAN TWIST

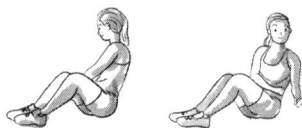

PREVIOUS BEST (WORKOUT 59)	REPS: _____	
SET 1	REPS: _____	(GOAL: 10-20 EACH SIDE)
SET 2	REPS: _____	(GOAL: 10-20 EACH SIDE)
SET 3	REPS: _____	(GOAL: 10-20 EACH SIDE)

4. PLANK

PREVIOUS BEST (WORKOUT 61)	TIME: _____	
SET 1	TIME: _____	(GOAL: 45-90 SECONDS)
SET 2	TIME: _____	(GOAL: 45-90 SECONDS)
SET 3	TIME: _____	(GOAL: 45-90 SECONDS)

SUPERSETS DONE TODAY (CIRCLE):
1   2   3   4

TODAY'S WORKOUT INTENSITY:
_____ / 10

Workout 65: Full Body Circuit

*Rest for **15-20 seconds** between each exercise, then rest for **1-2 minutes** after completing the entire circuit. Complete the full circuit **a total of 4-5 times.***

1. RUN IN PLACE

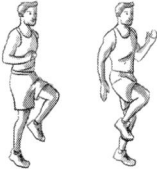

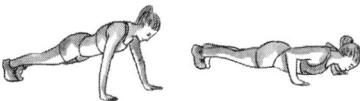

(Duration: 30 Seconds)

2. MOUNTAIN CLIMBER

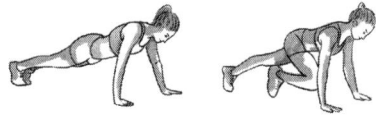

(Duration: 30 Seconds)

3. STARFISH CRUNCH

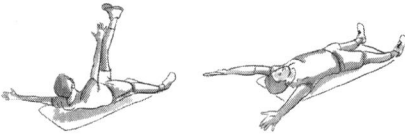

(Duration: 30 Seconds)

4. BICYCLE CRUNCH

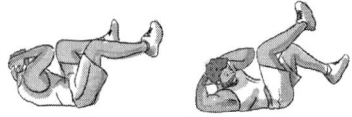

(Duration: 30 Seconds)

5. ALTERNATING LUNGE

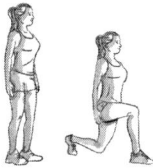

(Duration: 30 Seconds)

6. TOWEL SNATCH

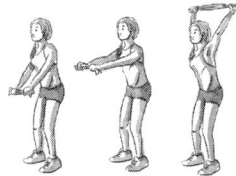

(Duration: 30 Seconds)

7. PUSH-UP

(Duration: 30 Seconds)

8. VERTICAL LEAP

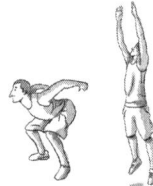

(Duration: 30 Seconds)

TODAY'S WORKOUT INTENSITY:

_____ / 10

<u>Congratulations!!!</u>

You've made it to the end of the journal and completed an INTENSE weightlifting regimen that has no doubt increased your strength, appearance, confidence, and ability to accomplish your goals.

For you to have gotten this far means you've earned a very serious congratulations. You need to celebrate because your willpower and confidence should be soaring through the roof.

You've gained lessons about yourself not many dare to approach. You've struggled with your own mind, body and heart and gained some serious control over them. You fully understand that you have the power in you to accomplish ANY goal you put your mind to.

That's so awesome.

You are a true WARRIOR.

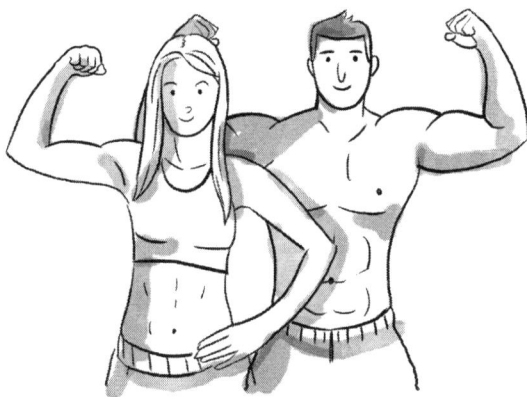

Note: We LOVE sharing stories of our users and what their lives looked like BEFORE using the journal compared to where they are NOW!

If you want to share your story with us, you can do so here:
habitnest.com/weightliftingtestimonial

Check-In

How has my life changed since I started this program?

_____

_____

_____

_____

What changes have I seen in my attitude?

_____

_____

_____

_____

What physical changes have I seen?

_____

_____

_____

_____

How do I feel about myself in general compared to when I started this program?

_____

_____

_____

_____

How do I see myself continuing to build on what I've learned and gained by doing this program?

_____

_____

_____

_____

- Fin -

So... What Now?

Although you should feel very accomplished for getting through this entire journal... know that you built this habit to *continually improve your life. Don't stop now. This is only the beginning.*

One huge factor to this is tracking your progress. Once you stop tracking, it makes it exponentially easier for you to skip having a consistent workout practice (due to the lack of accountability with yourself).

Remember: **Every single day in your life where you incorporate a strong foundation of fitness will automatically be a better day of your life.**

You only stand to gain from continuing this habit.

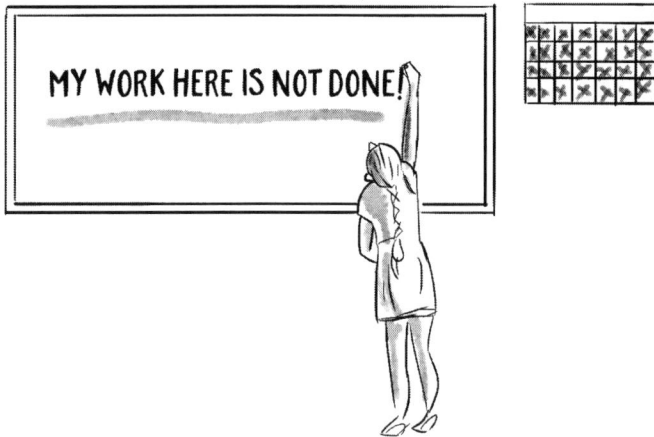

Continuing the Habit

The first question we get from users who finish the journal is 'what should I do now?' For that reason we created followup journal volumes to the *Weightlifting Gym Buddy Journal*!

If you think it'd be useful for you to continue growing with this practice, you can find out more here: **habitnest.com/weightliftingseries**

As of Fall 2019, we've launched new followup journals to the **Weightlifting Gym Buddy Journal**:

- The Weightlifting Gym Buddy Journal - Volume I
- **The Weightlifting Gym Buddy Journal - Volume II**
- **The Weightlifting Gym Buddy Journal - Volume III**
- **The Weight Training Tracker**

Volumes II and III of the journal gradually increase the difficulty of each workout as time goes on, helping to promote continual muscle development and introduce further variety to your workouts.

By the time you complete all three starting journals, you will have found which exercises have been most impactful for you and your progress. The final journal, *The Weight Training Tracker,* becomes a blank canvas for you to design your own workouts each day and follow along from there.

If you feel it would be helpful to continue this practice and tracking your progress, these are the tools for you.

You can get yours here!

habitnest.com/weightliftingseries

Shop Habit Nest Products

Lifestyle Products

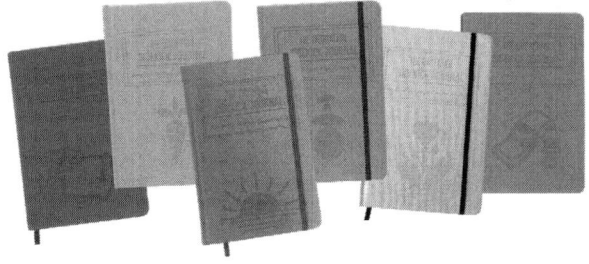

All of our lifestyle journals come with **daily content** (including Pro-Tips, Daily Challenges, Practical Resources, & more) to inspire you and give you bite-sized information to use along your journey. They also contain **daily questions aimed at holding you accountable** to ingraining that habit into your life.

The Morning Sidekick Journal Series

A set of guided morning planners that help you conquer your mornings and conquer your life. This complete 4-volume series covers one year of morning routines.

The Evening Routine & Sleep Sidekick Journal

Helps you to wind down your days peacefully, prepare for each next day, and get the most rejuvenating sleep of your life.

The Gratitude Sidekick Journal Series

A set of research-based journals that will help make an attitude of appreciation
a core part of who you are. There are 3 Volumes in total.

The Meditation Sidekick Journal

Built to give you all the tools you need to stay consistent with a meditation practice.

The Nutrition Sidekick Journal

Your nutrition tracker, informational guide, and coach, all in one.

The Budgeting Sidekick Journal Series

The most simple-yet-effective budgeting guide in the world, helping you find full clarity on your budgeting goals and to achieve financial freedom. Set spending goals, track your daily spending, and reconcile along the way. Contains two volumes, which cover well over a year of budgeting.

Fitness Products

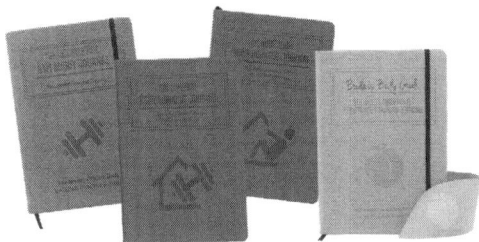

Our no-nonsense fitness books have fully guided fitness routines. No thinking required; just open the books and follow along.

The Weightlifting Gym Buddy Journal Series

A set of guided personal training programs aimed at helping you have the best workouts of your life. This complete 4-volume series covers one year of weightlifting workouts.

The Bodyweight / Dumbbell Home Workout Journals

Specifically focus on HOME workout programs that require minimal-to-no equipment to complete.

The Badass Body Goals Journal

An at-home-friendly fitness journal that focuses on HIIT and circuit workouts.
This journal comes with a full video guide you can play and follow along.

Other Products

The Habit Nest Daily Planner

Plan your day including your top priorities, smaller 5-minute tasks, and all your to-dos. Get optional suggestions for ways to start your mornings and end your evenings with as well.

George The Short-Necked Giraffe (Children's Book)

Follow along George's journey as he learns the hard way that fully accepting himself, exactly the way he is, is the only path to living his happiest life.

Shop all products here: **habitnest.com/store**

The Habit Nest Mobile App

The Habit Nest app offers a **digital representation of our journals**, with the benefit of improved tracking, varying ways to showcase content, and gamification, and more.

When Habit Nest was initially founded, it was supposed to be in mobile app form from the start.

As a team of three young founders with no outside funding to get a mobile app built, we started with paper journals that worked using the same concept,
which you're currently holding.

5 years and hundreds of thousands of journals sold later, we were finally able to create our mobile app and released it at the end of 2021.

We will always continue to print physical journals for every habit we release, only now, they'll also be put into the app so that everyone can experience our habit journeys in the way that suits them best.

If you're interested in seeing seeing whether the app is right for you,
feel free to see more at **habitnest.com/app**

With a lot of love,

**Mikey Ahdoot, Ari Banayan,
& Amir Atighehchi
Co-Founders of Habit Nest**

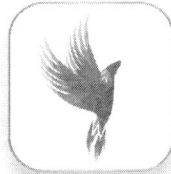

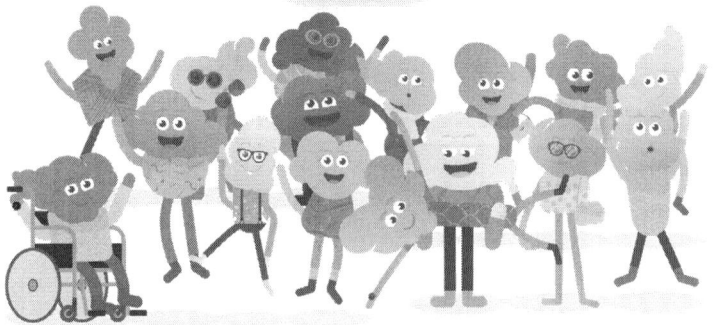

The Phoenixes Access Pass

We released *The Phoenixes* – Habit Nest's Special Access Pass – in 2022.

Anyone who purchases a Phoenix gets:

1. **Lifetime access** to the Habit Nest app.

2. Access to a **Learn2Earn system** we're building within the app, in which you will have chances to earn prizes/rewards for using our app to build better habits.

3. **First dibs** on new journal releases & our best discounts.

If you're interested in purchasing a Phoenix, visit:
https://habitnest.com/vip

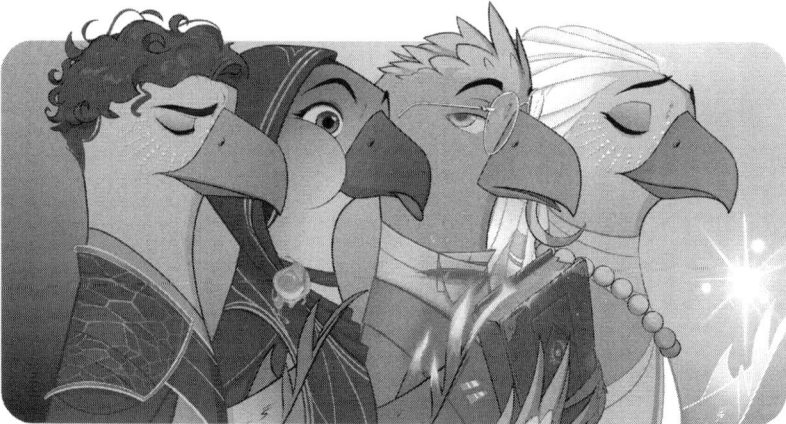

For more information, follow The Phoenixes on Twitter: **@thephoenixesnft**

Content Index

Workout Index

Workout Index

Ab Workouts

Bicycle Crunch

1. Lie flat with your lower back pressed to the ground. Place your hands behind your head slightly above your neck. Lift your shoulders into a crunch position.

2. Raise yours legs so that your thighs are perpendicular to the ground and your shins parallel to the ground.

3. Simultaneously, slowly go through a cycle pedal motion kicking forward with the right leg while pulling in the knee of the left leg.

4. Bring your right elbow close to your left knee by crunching to the side. Then crunch to the opposite side as you cycle your legs and bring your left elbow closer to your right knee.

5. Alternate sides.

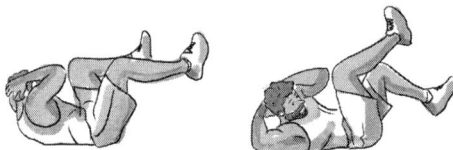

Starfish Crunch

1. Lie on your back with your arms and legs stretched out into an 'X' position.

2. In one movement, bring one arm straight up across your body while simultaneously lifting your opposing leg and lifting your head.

3. Attempt to touch one arm to your opposite ankle, or try to come as close as you can.

4. Alternate sides.

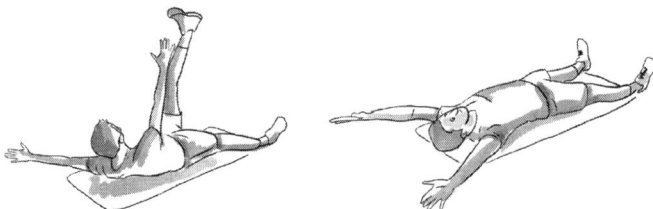

Ab Workouts

Leg Lift

1. Lie with your back flat on the floor (or on a bench) with your legs extended in front of you.

2. Place your hands to your sides with your palms facing down. To keep your hands down for support, you can place them under your glutes.

3. Keep your legs fully extended and as straight as possible (it's okay if your knees slightly bend). Hold the contraction at the top for a second.

4. Slowly lower your legs back down to the starting position.

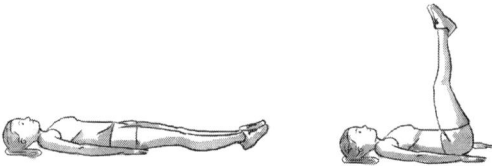

Hanging Leg Lift

1. Hang from a chin-up bar with both arms extended at arms length in top of you using either a wide grip or a medium grip. The legs should be straight down with the pelvis rolled slightly backwards. This will be your starting position.

2. Raise your legs until the torso makes a 90-degree angle with the legs. Hold for 0.5-1 seconds.

3. Repeat for the recommended amount of repetitions.

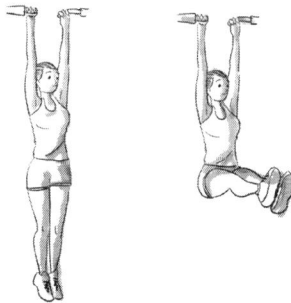

Ab Workouts

Kneeling Cable Crunch

Caution: Do not choose a weight that is too heavy. This can result in straining your lower back.

1. Find a cable station and attach a rope handle to the top pulley. Grasp the rope attachment at each end, and kneel down so your knees are bent at a 90° angle.

2. Your arms should be stretched over your head. Your palms should be facing each other when holding the rope and your hands should be placed next to your face.

3. Slightly flex your hips forward. There should be tension on the cable, and you should feel a stretch in your abs.

4. Keep your hips stationary, contract your abs, and crunch your chest towards your hips until your head is between your knees. Your elbows should be approaching the middle of your thighs. After reaching this point, hold the contraction for a second.

5. Slowly reverse back to the starting position. Keep as much tension in your abs during this whole movement.

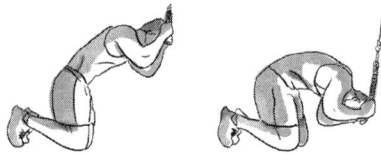

Plank

1. Place your forearms on the ground with your elbows aligned beneath your shoulders. Keep your arms parallel to your body at about shoulder-width distance. (You should be in a push-up position, only on your forearms rather than your hands).

2. Ground your toes into the floor and squeeze your glutes to stabilize your body. Be careful to not to lock or hyperextend your knees.

3. Neutralize your neck and spine by looking at a spot on the floor about a foot in front of your hands. Your head should be in line with your back. Contract your abdominals to keep yourself up and prevent your booty from sticking up.

4. Keep your back flat and hold the position for as long as possible without compromising form.

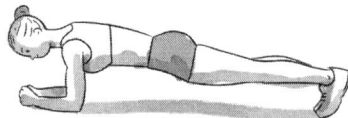

Russian Twist

1. Lie down on the floor placing your feet either under something that will not move or by having a partner hold them. Your legs should be bent at the knees.

2. Elevate your upper body so that it creates an imaginary V-shape with your thighs. Your arms should be fully extended in front of you perpendicular to your torso and with the hands clasped. This is the starting position.

3. Twist your torso to the right side until your arms are parallel with the floor while breathing out.

4. Hold the contraction for a second and move back to the starting position while breathing out. Now move to the opposite side performing the same techniques you applied to the right side.

5. Repeat for the recommended amount of repetitions.

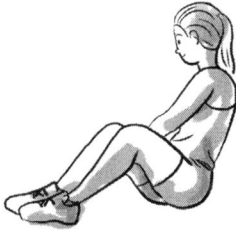 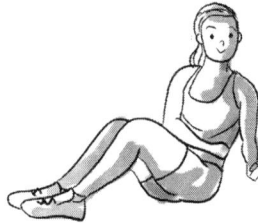

Back Workouts

Assisted Pull-Up

1. Securely set the pin on the desired weight. Unlike other machines, the **heavier** the weight you use, the **easier** this exercise will be (as the weight really serves as an assist, not resistance).

2. Stand on the platform, and grab the wide pull-up handles above your head. You can also do this on your knees.

3. Keep your abs engaged, spine neutral, and shoulders pressed down and back.

4. Pull yourself up as far as possible, making sure to keep your abs are engaged and your shoulders are pressed down and back. Simultaneously try to activate yours lats.

5. Slowly release yourself downwards until your arms are almost straight.

6. Repeat for the desired amount of reps.

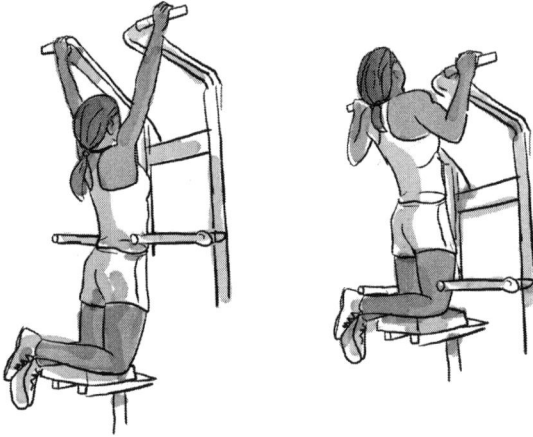

Bent Over Dumbbell Row

1. Find a flat bench and place a dumbbell on each side. Start by placing your right knee on top of the bench.

2. Bend your torso forward from your waist. Your upper body should be parallel to the ground. Place your right hand on the bench with your palm facing down, above where your knee is positioned. Place your left foot on the ground beside the bench.

3. Use your left hand to pick up the dumbbell with an overhand grip (your palm should be facing your torso). Keep your arm fully extended and make sure to keep your lower back straight.

4. Keep your elbow close to your side while you pull the weight straight up towards your chest. As you pull the weight up, concentrate on squeezing your back muscles and shoulder blades (you should feel a contraction in your back muscles).

5. Slowly lower the weight straight down with control.

6. Alternate sides.

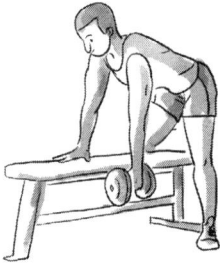 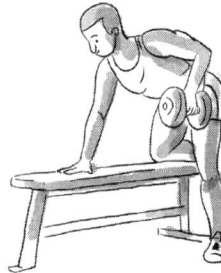

Back Workouts

Close Grip Cable Row

Caution: Avoid swinging your torso back and forth. This can result in a lower back injury.

1. Attach a V-bar to the low pulley on a seated row machine. When gripping the V-bar, your palms should be facing each other.

2. Sit down on the machine and place your feet on the front platform with your knees slightly bent.

3. Grab the V-bar handles, lean over, and keep your back upright with your shoulders back. Your back should be slightly arched with your chest sticking out. As you hold the bar in front of you, you should you should notice a stretch in your lats.

4. Keep your torso stationary and your elbows tucked in as you pull the handles back towards your torso. You should be squeezing your back muscles and holding that contraction for a second.

5. Slowly return the weight to starting position by releasing your shoulder blades back down.

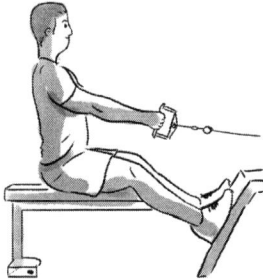

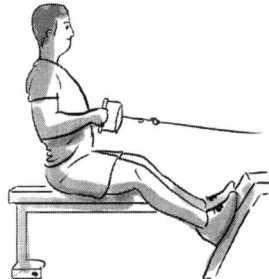

Back Workouts

Lat Pulldown (Regular, Reverse-Grip, Close-Grip)

1. Attach a wide-grip handle to the lat pulldown machine. Adjust the knee pad of the machine to fit your height to prevent your lower body from moving while performing this movement.

2. For a regular lat pulldown, grasp the bar with an overhand grip with your arms at the end of the flat bar.

   For a reverse-grip lat pulldown, use an underhand grip and your palms facing your body.

   For a close grip, your hands should be positioned shoulder-width apart.

3. Extend both arms up above you while holding the bar. Keep your back upright, create a slight curvature in your lower back, and stick out your chest.

4. Keep your torso stationary and pull the bar down towards your body by drawing your shoulder blades and upper arms down and back. Squeeze your back muscles during this movement.

5. Slowly raise the bar in a controlled motion back to the starting position. Your arms should be fully extended and your lats fully stretched.

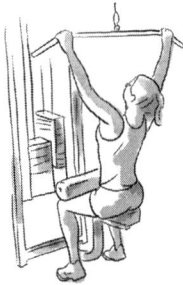 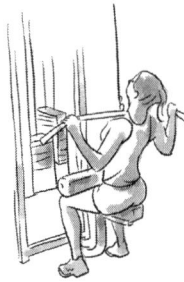

Regular-Grip

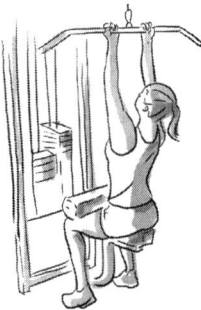 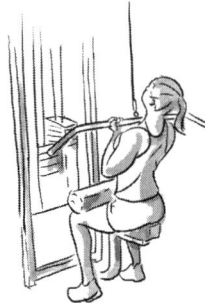

Reverse-Grip

Back Workouts

Pull-Up

1. Grasp the pull bar with a grip wider than your shoulder-width.

2. Take a deep breath and depress the shoulder blades. Drive your elbows straight down to the floor to pull yourself up. Simultaneously try to activate yours lats.

3. Pull your chin towards the bar until your lats are fully contracted. Slowly lower yourself back to the starting position and repeat. Try to do this motion slowly.

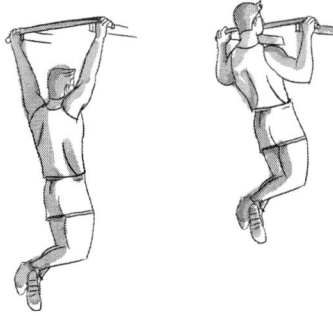

Straight Arm Pulldown

1. Attach a wide bar at your shoulder-level on the pulley of the pulldown machine. Grab the bar with an overhand grip with your palms facing downward, and make sure your grip is wider than your shoulder-width.

2. Take a couple steps back and make sure your feet are shoulder-width apart. Slightly hinge at the waist so that your torso is leaning forward. Keep your arms fully extended so that they're parallel to the ground. Your arms can have a slight bend at the elbow.

3. Pull the bar down while keeping your arms straight. Continue pulling down until your hands are beside your thighs; you should feel a contraction in your lats.

4. Reverse this movement while keeping your arms fully straight.

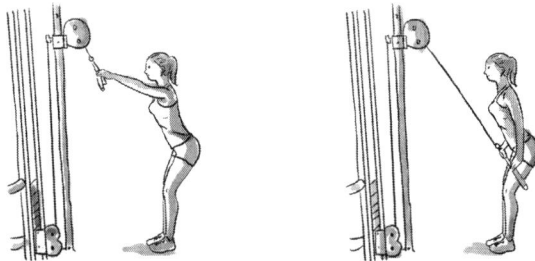

T-Bar Row

1. Load an appropriate weight onto the end of the T-bar.

2. Stand over the bar so that it's in between your legs and your chest is resting on the pad. Keep your back flat and make sure you have a firm grip on each side of the V-grip handle.

3. Remove the bar from the rest. Keep your chest up, your hips back, and your feet wider than shoulder-width apart. Lead the movement with your back, your arms should follow. The focus should not be on the angle of your arms, but on the contraction of your back.

4. After your back reaches its maximum contraction and your shoulder blades are retracted, slowly let the weight of the bar pull your shoulder blades down to stretch your back.

5. Let your arms follow naturally until the T-bar is returned to its starting position.

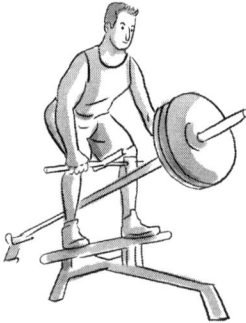

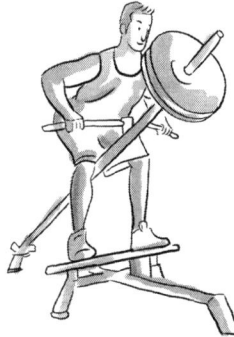

Back Workouts

Upper Back Rope Pull

1. Stand in front of a medium-height rotating pulley and grab each side of the rope attachment.

2. Step back away from the machine until your arms are fully extended in front of you.

3. Your feet should be slightly wider than shoulder width apart and with a soft bend in your knees.

4. Brace core 3and drive elbows past back, while pulling the rope handles slightly outside of your ears.

5. Hold and contract shoulder blades together.

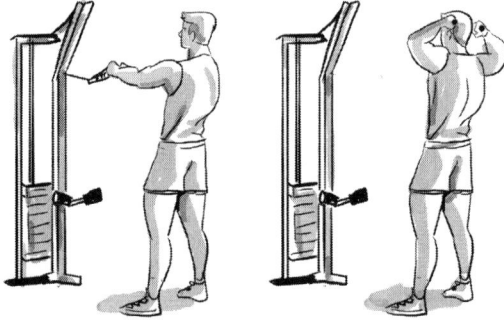

Bicep Workouts

Concentration Curl

1. Sit at the end of a bench and place one dumbbell in front of you between your legs. Keep your legs spread apart, your knees bent, your back straight, and your feet on the ground.

2. Use your right arm to pick up the dumbbell. Place the back of your arm against the inside of your same-sided thigh.

3. Begin with the the palm of your hand facing away from your thigh. Keep your arm extended and the dumbbell slightly above the ground.

4. Make sure that your upper arm remains stationary as you contract your biceps and curl the dumbbell toward your opposite-sided pec. Continue the movement until the dumbbell is at shoulder-level. Remember, only the forearms should move.

5. Slowly begin to lower the dumbbell back to its starting position. Avoid swinging motions at all times.

6. Perform all reps using the same arm, then repeat this movement with your other arm.

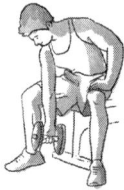

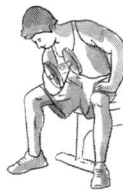

Dumbbell Hammer Curl

1. Stand upright with your feet shoulder-width apart. Hold a dumbbell in each hand with your arms extended along your sides. Your elbows should be tucked in close to your torso and your palms should be facing your torso.

2. Keep your upper arm stationary as you contract your biceps and curl the dumbbells directly upward. Continue to raise the dumbbells until your biceps are fully contracted and the dumbbell is at shoulder-level. Focus on only moving your forearm.

3. After a brief pause, slowly begin to lower the dumbbells back down to the starting position.

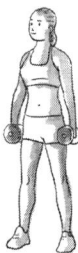

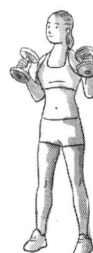

Bicep Workouts

Overhead Cable Curl

1. To begin, set a weight that is comfortable on each side of the pulley machine. Make sure the weight selected is equal on each side.

2. Adjust the height of the pulleys on each side so that they're positioned higher than shoulder height.

3. Stand in the middle of both sides and use an underhand grip to grab each handle. Your arms should be fully extended to each side and parallel to the ground. Your palms should be facing upward and your feet positioned shoulder-width apart.

4. Keep your elbows in a fixed position as you slowly squeeze your biceps and curl your hands toward your shoulders. You should be squeezing in your biceps until your forearms and biceps touch.

5. Lower your forearms back to the starting position while keeping your entire body stationary.

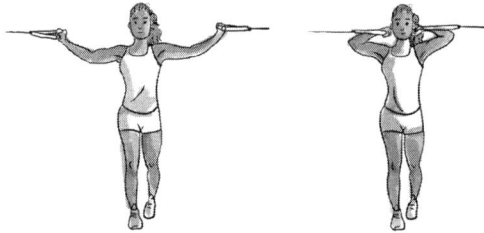

Preacher Curl

1. To perform this movement, you will need a preacher bench and an EZ bar. Load your desired weight onto the bar and adjust the seat on the preacher bench so that your upper arms sit comfortably on the padding when you're seated.

2. Grab the EZ bar using an underhand grip with your palms facing upward. Lift the EZ bar to shoulder height.

3. As you inhale, slowly lower the bar until your upper arms are extended and your biceps are fully stretched.

4. As you exhale, curl the bar up until your biceps are fully contracted and the bar is at your shoulder height. Try to squeeze your biceps tightly and hold this position for a second if you can.

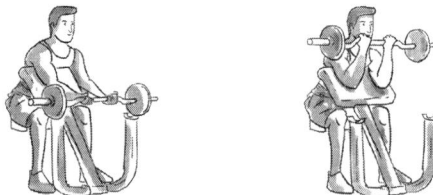

Rope Hammer Curl

1. Hook a rope attachment to the low pulley and stand facing the machine about one foot away from it.

2. Grasp the rope with your palms facing inward. Make sure you stand up straight, maintain the natural arch of your back, and keep your torso stationary.

3. Start with your elbows tucked in by your side. Using your biceps, pull your arms up until your forearms touch your biceps. Only your forearms should move, not your upper arms. Remember to keep your elbows tucked in by your sides and your upper arms stationary.

4. Slowly lower the rope back to the starting position.

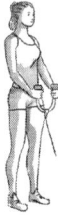

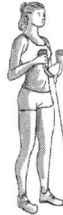

Seated Dumbbell Curl

1. Sit on a bench with a back support and place your feet shoulder-width apart. Take a deep breath before beginning. Sit up straight with a dumbbell in each hand at arm's length. Keep your elbows close to your torso and rotate the palms of your hands until they are facing inward.

2. Curl the weights while contracting your biceps so that your palms are facing backwards. Continue to raise the dumbbells until your biceps are fully contracted and the dumbbells are at shoulder-level. Try to hold the contracted position for a brief pause as you squeeze your biceps. Make sure to keep your upper arms and elbows stationary through the movement; your forearms should be the only part moving during this exercise.

3. Slowly begin to lower the dumbbells back to the starting position.

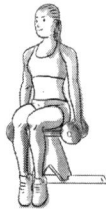

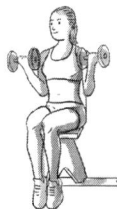

Bicep Workouts

Underhand Cable Curl

1. Attach a wide bar or individual handles to a cable tower.

2. Grasp the attachment(s) with a wide underhand grip. With your arms straight, your core tight and a neutral spine.

3. Keeping the elbows at your sides and your head forward, curl the bar up to your chest.

4. Lower the bar under control. Do not let your upper back round over - consciously pull your shoulder blades together to provide a stable base for your arms to pull from.

5. Do not swing - keep your core tight and a neutral spine.

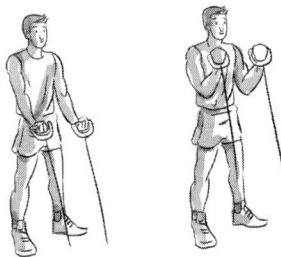

Zottman Curl

1. Stand upright with a dumbbell in each of your hands at arm's length. Your elbows should be tucked in close to your torso. Make sure your palms are facing your body before beginning the movement.

2. Contract your biceps as you curl the dumbbells upward; only your forearms should be moving. As you curl up, rotate your wrists so that your palms are facing upward, like in an underhand grip. Continue this movement until the dumbbells are at your shoulder-level.

3. Try to hold the contracted position for a second while sweeping your biceps. Then, in the contracted position, rotate your wrists again until you your palms are facing down, like in an overhand grip.

4. With this overhand grip, slowly lower the dumbbells back down.

5. As the dumbbells approach your thighs, rotate your wrists to return to your original grip with your palms facing inward towards your body.

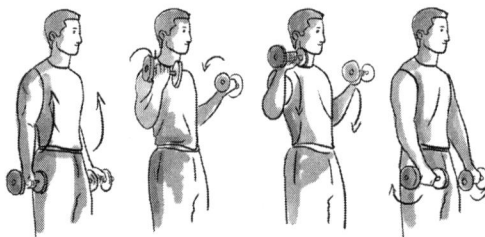

Chest Workouts

Cable Crossover

1. Place the pulleys on a high position above your head and select the same resistance for each side's handle.

2. Stand between both pulleys and move one foot slightly forward. With an overhand grip, pull your arms together in front of you. Your torso should be leaning slightly forward from your waist.

3. With a slight bend in your elbows, extend your arms into a wide arc until you feel a stretch in your chest. Your arms and torso should remain stationary.

4. Using the same arc of motion, return your arms back to the starting position.

5. Hold for a second at the starting position and repeat the movement.

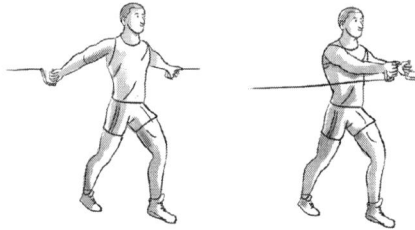

Chest Fly w/ Machine

1. Sit with your back flat against the pad and your feet flat on the ground; adjust the seat if necessary.

2. With your arms positioned parallel to the ground, grasp the handles. Adjust the machine to fit your size.

3. Keeping your elbows slightly bent, slowly push the handles together as you squeeze the middle of your chest and contract your pectorals.

4. Slowly return handles to the starting position until your chest muscles are fully stretched

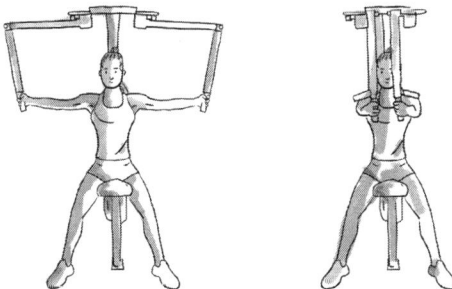

Chest Workouts

Decline Bench Press

Caution: In order to protect yourself, it is best to have a spotter help you.

1. Start by securing your legs under the brace at the bottom of the decline bench and lie down.

2. Using an overhand medium-width grip, lift the bar from the rack and hold it straight over your chest with your arms full extended. Your arms should be perpendicular to the ground.

3. As you inhale, lower the bar toward your chest until your elbows reach a 90° angle.

4. Pause for a second, then use your chest muscles to push the bar back up to the starting position as you exhale. Lock your arms and squeeze your chest in at the contracted position. Hold for a second and then start to lower the bar down slowly.

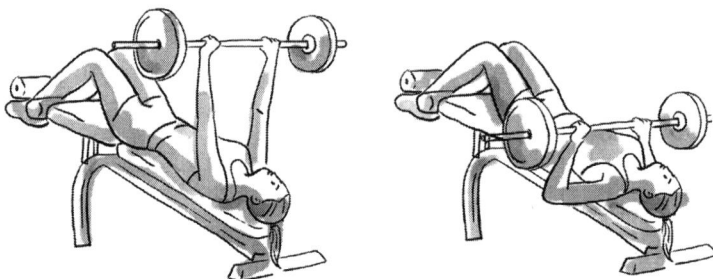

Flat Bench Press

Caution: In order to protect yourself, it is best to have a spotter help you.

1. Start by lying back on a flat bench. Use an overhand grip that is wider than your shoulder-width to lift the bar from the rack. Hold it directly above you with your arms fully extended.

2. Inhale and begin lowering the bar toward your chest until your elbow creates a 90° angle.

3. After a brief pause, push the bar back to the starting position as you exhale. Focus on using your chest muscles to push up the bar.

4. Lock your arms and squeeze your chest in the contracted position at the top of the motion. Hold for a second and then slowly begin lowering the bar.

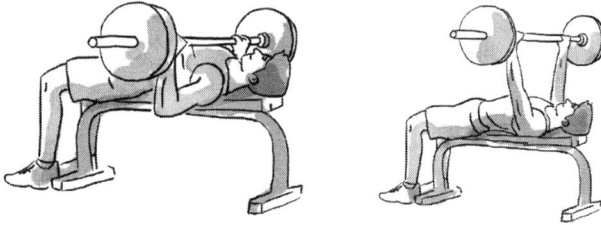

Incline Dumbbell Fly

1. Pick up the dumbbells and grip them so that so your palms are facing inward. Lie back on an incline bench angled at about 30 degrees, and rest the dumbbells on your hip crease.

2. Press the dumbbells out and over you so that your arms are fully extended. Rotate your wrists so that your palms are facing each other.

3. Slightly retract your shoulder blades, unlock your elbows, and slowly lower the dumbbells laterally to create a wide arc while maintaining the angle at your elbow. You should feel stretch in your chest.

4. Once the dumbbells reach your chest level, reverse the movement while trying not to let the dumbbells touch.

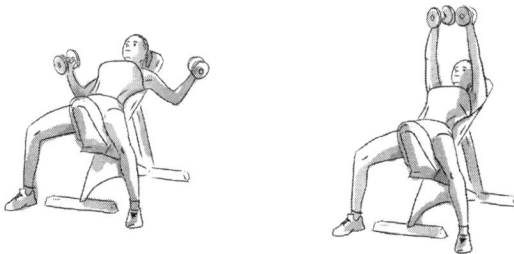

Chest Workouts

Incline Dumbbell Press

1. Lie back on an incline bench with a dumbbell in each hand atop your thighs. The palms of your hands will be facing each other.

2. Then, using your thighs to help push the dumbbells up, lift the dumbbells one at a time so that you can hold them at shoulder-width.

3. Once you have the dumbbells raised to shoulder-width, rotate your wrists forward so that the palms of your hands are facing away from you. This will be your starting position.

4. Be sure to keep full control of the dumbbells at all times. Then, breathe out and push the dumbbells up with your chest.

5. Lock your arms at the top, hold for a second, and then start slowly lowering the weight. Note: Ideally, lowering the weights should take about twice as long as raising them.

6. Repeat the movement for the prescribed number of repetitions.

7. When you are done, place the dumbbells back on your thighs and then on the floor. This is the safest manner to release the dumbbells.

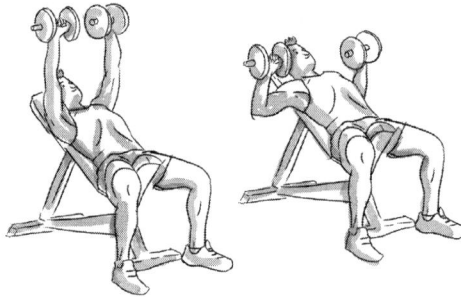

High to Low Cable Fly

1. Move the pulleys to the highest position and select the same resistance for each D-handle.

2. Stand between both pulleys with your arms extended out to your sides. Grasp both handles with an overhand grip while keeping your feet aligned with the pulleys.

3. Remaining upright and keeping a slight bend in your elbows, pull your arms close together in front of your body.

4. After a pause at the peak contraction, return your arms back to the starting position.

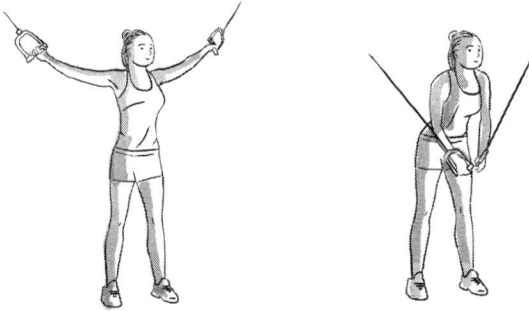

Low to High Cable Fly

1. Place the pulleys at the lowest position and select the same resistance level for each one.

2. Stand between both pulleys with your arms extended out to your sides. Grasp both handles with an underhand grip so that your palms are facing forward and move one foot forward.

3. Start with your hands below your waist and your arms fully extended.

4. Keep a slight bend in your elbows as you raise your arms upward and towards the middle of your torso. Make sure that you are flexing your chest. Your hands should end up being directly in front of your chest.

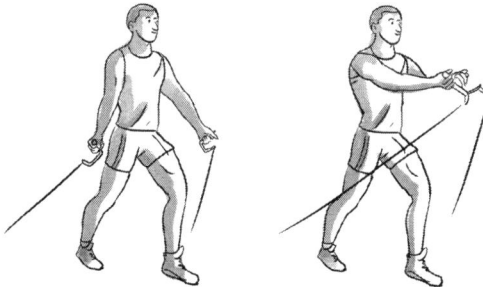

Chest Workouts

Flat Bench Dumbbell Press

1. Lie down on a flat bench with a dumbbell in each hand resting on top of your thighs. The palms of your hands will be facing each other.

2. Then, using your thighs to help raise the dumbbells up, lift the dumbbells one at a time so that you can hold them in front of you at shoulder width.

3. Once at shoulder width, rotate your wrists forward so that the palms of your hands are facing away from you. The dumbbells should be just to the sides of your chest, with your upper arm and forearm creating a 90 degree angle.

4. Use your chest to push the dumbbells up. Lock your arms at the top of the lift and squeeze your chest, hold for a second and then begin coming down slowly.

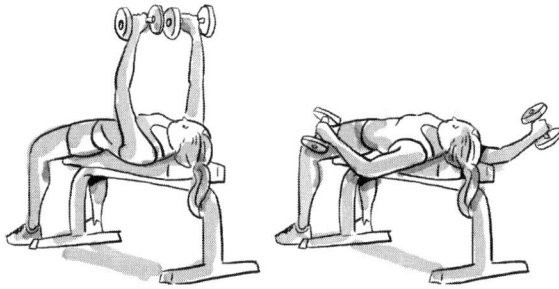

Flat Bench Dumbbell Fly

1. Pick up the dumbbells, one in each hand, with your palms facing inward. Sit down on a flat bench and rest the dumbbells on your thighs.

2. Before laying down, lift the dumbbells in front of you at shoulder width keeping your palms facing each other. To get into position, lay back and keep the dumbbells close to your chest.

3. When you're ready, press the dumbbells out and above you so that your arms are fully extended.

4. Slightly retract your shoulder blades, unlock your elbows, and slowly lower the dumbbells laterally to create a wide arc while maintaining the angle at your elbow. You should feel stretch in your chest.

5. Once the dumbbells reach your chest level, reverse the movement while trying not to let the dumbbells touch.

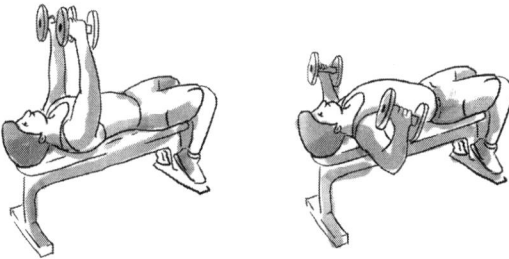

Push-Up

1. Lie on the ground face down and place your hands shoulder width apart. Push your body off the ground through your hands while keeping your back as straight as possible.

2. Lower yourself back down until your chest nearly touches the ground as you inhale.

3. Exhale and press your upper body back up to the starting position while squeezing your chest, arms, and abdominal muscles.

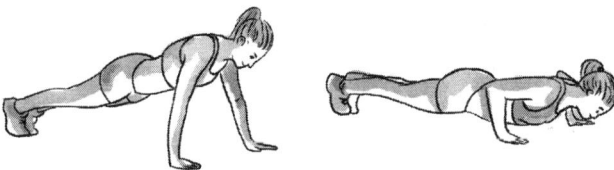

Circuit Workouts

Alternating Lunge

Caution: This movement requires a great deal of balance so if you lack balance or are suffering from an injury that affects your balance, hold on to a fixed object while completing this movement.

1. Stand with your torso upright and your hands by your sides.

2. Step forward with your right foot about 2 feet in front of you while lowering your upper body and maintaining your balance. Leave your left foot stationary behind you.

3. Squat down through your hips. Do not allow your front knee to extend beyond your toes as you lower yourself. Keep your front shin perpendicular to the ground.

4. Using mainly the heel of your foot, drive yourself back up to the starting position.

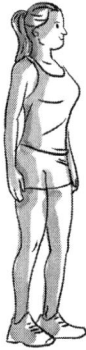

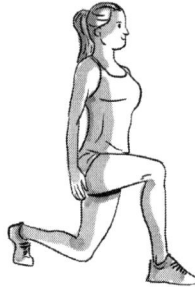

5. Alternate sides.

Air Squat

1. Stand upright with your feet a little wider than hip-width apart and your toes turned slightly out. If you can, engage your abdominal muscles and broaden your chest by gently pulling your shoulder blades in toward each other.

2. Bend your knees slowly, pushing your glutes and hips out and down behind you as if you're sitting down on a chair. Keep your head and shoulders aligned with your knees and your knees aligned with your ankles.

3. Lower your body until your thighs are parallel to the ground. Keep your knees alined with your toes (without surpassing them) as you lower yourself as straight down as possible. You can raise your arms up and in front of you (no higher than parallel to the ground) as you lower your body.

4. Straighten your legs to come up and squeeze your glutes as you approach the starting position.

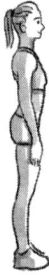

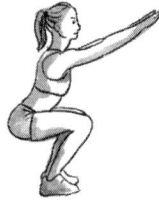

Burpee

1. Stand straight upright with both of your arms fully extended above your head.

2. Bring both hands to the ground in front of you and extend both legs straight behind you.

3. Jump or step your feet back to your hands.

4. Stand straight up and jump with your arms fully extended toward the ceiling.

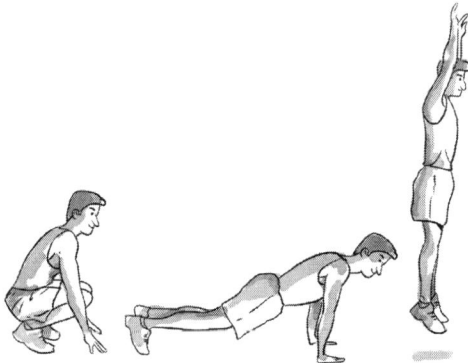

Circuit Workouts

Crunch

1. Lie on your back with your knees bent and feet resting flat on the ground hip-width apart.

2. Place your hands behind your head so that your thumbs are behind your ears.

3. Hold your elbows out to the sides and slightly tilted inward.

4. Slightly tilt your chin down, leaving a few inches of space between your chin and your chest.

5. Gently pull your abdominals inward.

6. Curl up and forward so that your head, neck, and shoulder blades lift off the ground.

7. Hold for a second at the top of the movement and then slowly lower yourself back down.

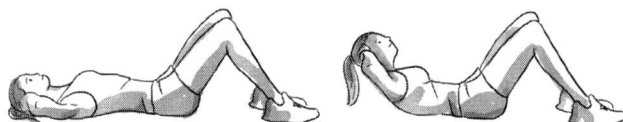

High Knee

1. Stand with your feet about shoulder-width apart.

2. Lift one leg as you drive your knee up toward your chest and raise your opposite arm. Slightly arch or round your lower back to keep your pelvis stationary and reduce strain on your back.

3. Quickly place your foot back on the ground.

4. Bring your opposite leg upward in the same motion, driving your knee to your chest, while raising your opposite arm. (This movement is essentially running in place to increase your heart rate.)

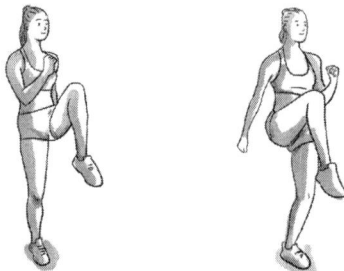

5. Alternate sides.

Circuit Workouts

Jump

1. Bend at the knees.

2. Jump in the air as high as you can!

3. Land softly on your feet.

4. Repeat.

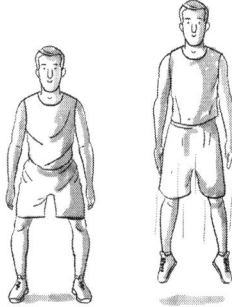

Jumping Jack

1. Stand with your feet together, knees slightly bent, and arms to your sides.

2. Jump while raising your arms and separating your legs. Land on your forefoot with your legs apart and arms overhead.

3. Jump again while lower your arms and returning your legs to midline. Land on your forefoot with your arms and legs in their original position and repeat.

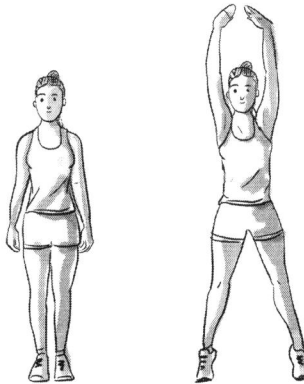

Circuit Workouts

Mountain Climber

1. Get in a push-up or plank position. Keep your abdominal muscles tight and your body straight while holding yourself off the floor.

2. Pull your right knee into your chest. Make sure that your body doesn't come out of its push-up or plank position. Keep your spine in a straight line and don't let your head slump. Having core body stability is very crucial for this movement.

3. Quickly place your right leg back down while simultaneously switching legs and pulling your left knee into your chest. Make sure that at the same time you push your right leg back, you pull your left knee into your chest using the same form. (This movement is essentially running in place while maintaining a straight and aligned body.)

4. Alternate sides.

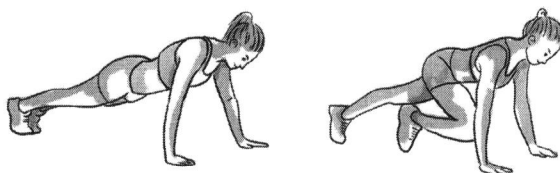

Prayer

1. Stand upright with your knees slightly bent.

2. Place your hands together in a praying position in front of your chest. Your elbows should be pointing out to your sides and your fingers pointing ahead of you while pushing tightly against each other.

3. Slowly move your hands outward away from your body so that your arms fully extend while still positioned together and pushing tightly against each other.

4. To feel this movement to its highest extent, you want to be pushing your hands together as tightly as you possible. You can try putting a 5 or 10 pound weighted plate between your hands to increase the difficulty.

5. Bring your wrists back in toward your chest.

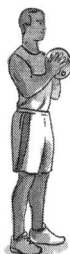
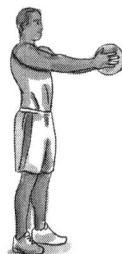

Run In Place

1. Stand with your feet about shoulder-width apart.

2. Lift one foot off the ground by bending at the knee and repeat the motion with alternating legs.

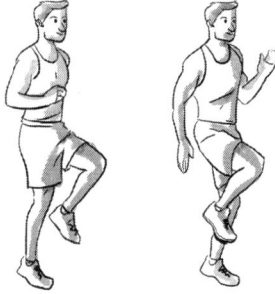

Side Plank

1. Lie down on your right side with your legs straight.

2. Prop yourself up with your right forearm so that your body forms a diagonal line.

3. Rest your left hand on your hip.

4. Brace your abdominal muscles and core.

5. Split the time between both sides of your body.

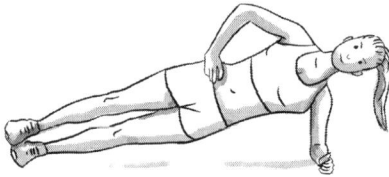

Circuit Workouts

Towel Pull

1. Grab a towel or t-shirt, hold it in both hands, and stand in a squat position.

2. Hold the towel out in front of you with your arms extended, and pull on both sides of the t-shirt or towel as hard, as you can as if you were trying to rip it.

3. As you continue to try to rip the towel or t-shirt, slowly bring your elbows backwards as if you were trying to squeeze your shoulder blades together.

4. When your hands get as close to your chest as possible, slowly return to the starting position and repeat until the set is complete. Remember to KEEP trying to rip the towel throughout the entire exercise.

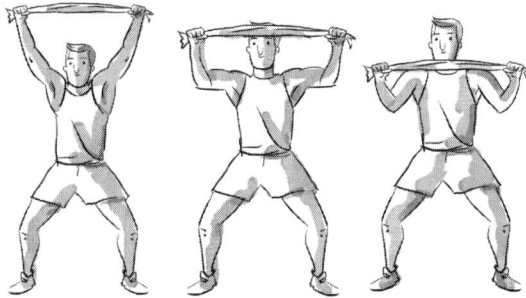

Towel Snatch

1. While holding a towel or t-shirt, get into a squat position with your feet wider than shoulder-width apart.

2. Hold the towel out in front of your body with your arms fully extended in front of you.

3. Spread your arms as if you are attempting to rip the towel in half.

4. While maintaining the squeeze of trying to rip the towel and keeping your arms straight, raise the towel up above your head and then lower it back down to the starting position.

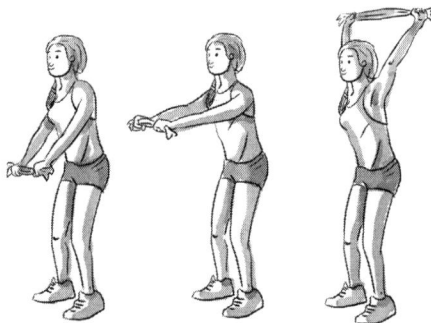

Vertical Leap

1. Sit in a deep squat position with your weight in your heels and your booty as far back as possible.

2. Using your arms for momentum, jump up as high as you can while extending your arms to the ceiling.

3. Land in the same seated squat position that you started in.

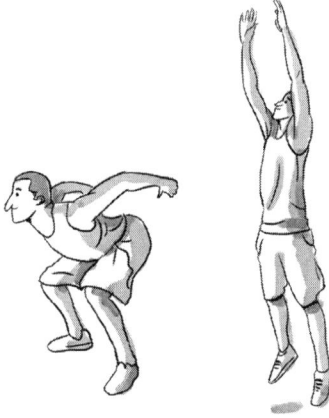

Forearm Workouts

Barbell Twist-Up

1. Stand upright and hold a barbell behind your back at the height of your glutes. Your arms should be fully extended with your hands placed shoulder-width apart and your palms facing the ground in overhand grip.

2. Keep your feet at shoulder-width apart and slowly elevate the barbell by curling your wrist in a semicircular motion toward the ceiling. Your wrists should be the only part moving.

3. Hold this position for a second then lower the barbell back down.

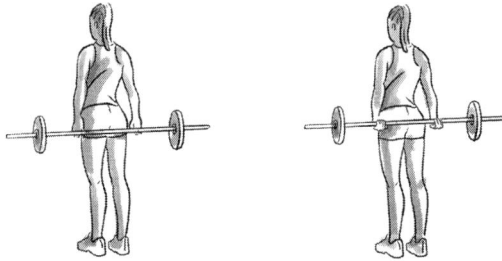

Dumbbell Twist-Up

1. Stand upright and hold two heavy dumbbells behind your back at the height of your glutes. Your arms should be fully extended with your hands placed shoulder-width apart and your palms facing the ground in overhand grip.

2. Keep your feet at shoulder-width apart and slowly elevate the barbell by curling your wrist in a semicircular motion toward the ceiling. Your wrists should be the only part moving.

3. Hold this position for a second then lower the barbell back down towards your fingertips.

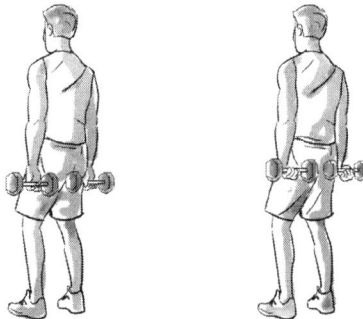

Farmer's Walk

1. Firmly grip two dumbbells from a dumbbell rack and lift them up, allowing your arms to then fall by your sides.

2. Walk around with your head facing forward and bracing your core until you cannot safely hold the dumbbells any longer.

3. Safely return the dumbbells to the rack when you are near failure. Be careful not to hold them for too long on this exercise as you can injure yourself easily by dropping them.

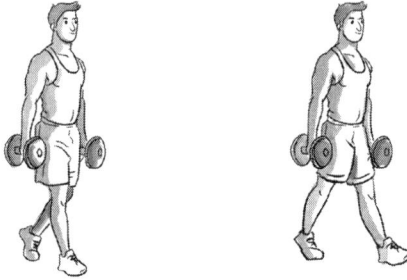

Pull-Up Bar Hang

1. Grip a pull-up bar with your palms facing away from your face.

2. Let your arms hang straight up and hold on for as long as you can. A good long-term target for this to build up to is 90 seconds - 120 seconds of hanging.

3. Let go once your grip gives out.

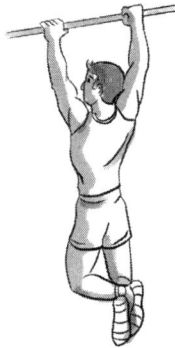

Forearm Workouts

Reverse Grip Dumbbell Curl

1. Grab a dumbbell in each hand and stand shoulder-width apart with your palms facing your body.

2. Without moving your elbows, lift the dumbbells in a curling motion towards the ceiling, while keeping your palms facing your body. It's just like doing a bicep curl with your hands facing the opposite direction.

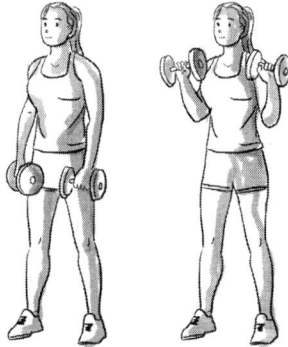

Reverse Grip EZ Bar Curl

1. Sit at a preacher curl bench. Select an EZ bar and grasp it with your palms facing downward at around shoulder-width apart.

2. Rest your elbows on the pad. Keep your upper arms stationary while slowly curling the bar up.

3. Do not pause, then slowly lower the weight back to the starting position.

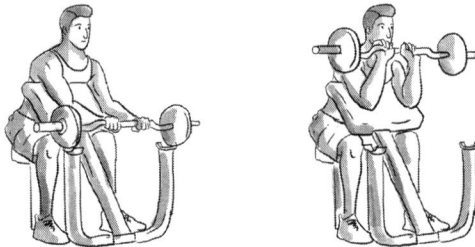

Leg Workouts

Leg Press

1. Using the leg press machine, sit down with your back and head against the padded support and place your feet on the footplate. Your feet should be approximately shoulder-width apart and aligned with your hips.

2. Unlock the safety bars holding the platform and press the platform all the way up until your legs are fully extended without locking your knees. Grasp the handles during the movement.

3. Slowly lower the platform until your thighs and calves create a 90° angle.

4. Drive the heels of your feet into the platform and press up using your quadriceps.

5. When complete, ensure to lock the safety pins properly and lock the safety bars.

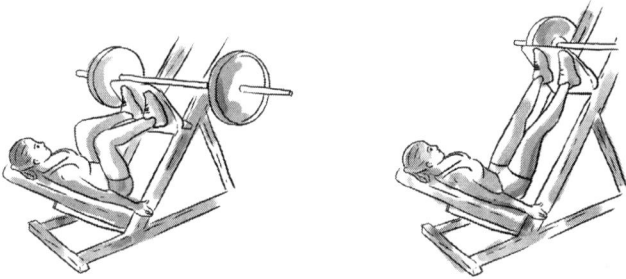

Leg Workouts

Deadlift

1. Stand upright with the barbell centered over your feet. Keep your feet hip-width apart and your toes slightly pointed outward. Hinge at your hips and use an overhand grip to grasp the bar at shoulder-width so that your shoulder blades can elongate.

2. Lower your hips and bend your knees until your shins come into contact with the bar. Look forward while keeping your chest up and your back arched. Drive through your heels to lift the weight upward.

3. After the bar passes your knees, pull it upward as you raise your chest and, thus, straightening your back. You should be pulling your shoulder blades together as you drive your hips forward into the bar. Make sure that you lock your hips and knees, move your booty back, and fire your glutes as you stand up with the bar (this movement comes from your hips, not your knees).

4. Unlock your hips and knees so that you can lower the bar by hinging your hips back down. Bend your knees after the bar passes them and use your hips to guide the bar to the ground. The bar should land centered over your feet at the starting position.

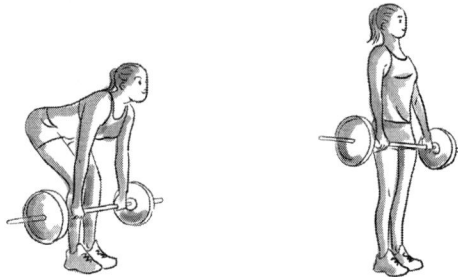

Barbell Squat

1. Find a squat rack and set the height of the bar slightly beneath your shoulders. Stand with your feet at about hip-width apart. Step up to the bar, move under it, and grip it with an overhand grip. The barbell should be supported on top of your traps.

2. Your chest should be up and your head facing forward. Once the bar is on your back, stand up, flex your core, tighten your glutes, and step away from the rack.

3. Begin squatting by lowering yourself until your legs reach a 90° angle and your thighs are parallel to the ground. Your knees will move forward, but ensure that they stay aligned with your feet.

4. While keeping your torso upright, drive your heels into the ground to push yourself back up.

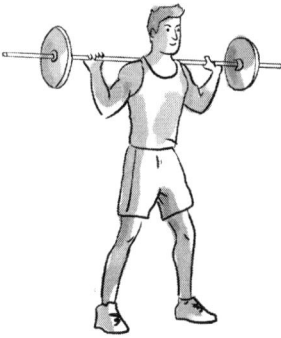

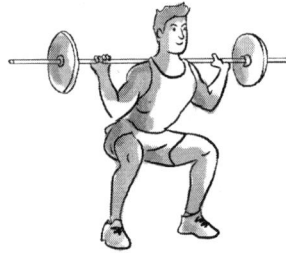

Leg Workouts

Hack Squat

1. Place the back of your torso against the pad of the machine and position your shoulders under the shoulder pads.

2. Place your feet shoulder-width apart with your toes slightly pointed outwards. Extend your legs, place your hands on the side handles, and unlock the safety handles. Make sure your back remains on the pad at all times.

3. Slowly begin to lower the unit by bending your knees. Keep your head up and maintain straight posture. Continue to lower the weight until you create a 90° angle, or slightly less, between your thighs and calves. Your knees should not move beyond your toes.

4. Lift the weight by driving your heels into the floor as you straighten your legs again.

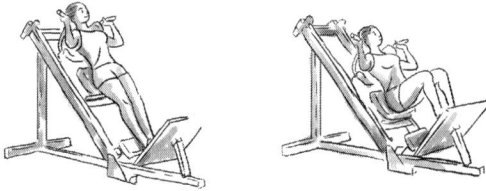

Quad Extension

1. Sit on the leg extension machine with your back agains the pad. Your legs should be under the padded lever and your feet pointing forward.

2. Adjust the pad so that it's placed above your feet and not at your shins. Your legs should create a 90° angle between your thighs and calves. Grasp the handles on the sides of the machine for support.

3. Using your quadriceps, extend your calves all the way out so that they align with your thighs. Grasp the handles to ensure your body remains stationary.

4. Hold for a second then slowly begin to lower the weight back down.

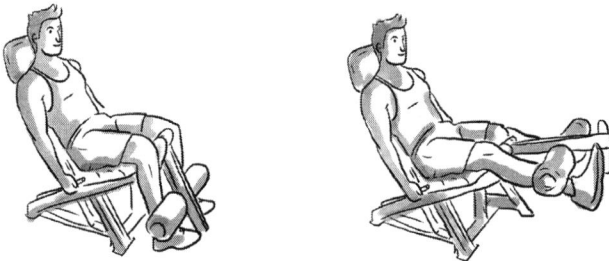

Hamstring Extension

1. Sit on the machine with your back against the pad. Adjust the leg pad so it rests against your ankles.

2. Secure the lap pad against your thighs, right above your knees. Grasp the handles on the machine to assist you in pointing your toes straight (flexing your feet).

3. Grasp the handles for support and flex your knees as you curl the weight back as far as possible toward the back of your thighs. Keep your torso stationary at all times and squeeze your hamstrings once you have moved the weight as far back as you can.

4. After a second, slowly return the weight to the starting position.

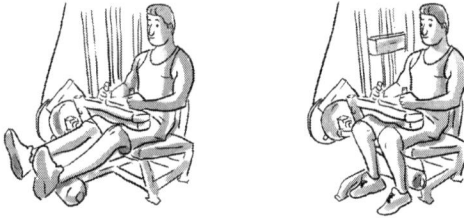

Weighted Lunge

Caution: This movement requires a great deal of balance, so if you lack balance or are suffering from an injury that affects your balance, use your own bodyweight while holding on to a fixed object.

1. Stand with your torso upright and hold one dumbbell in each hand at arm's length.

2. Step forward with your right foot (about 2 feet or so) as you lower your body down and squat through your hips. Make sure that your left foot remains stationary and that you are maintaining your balance. Do not allow your right knee to move beyond your toes as you come down. Keep your front shin perpendicular to the ground.

3. Using mainly the heel of your foot, drive yourself back up to the starting position.

4. Repeat the movement for your left leg.

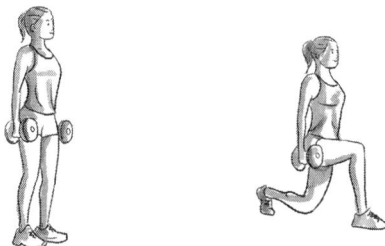

Leg Workouts

Calf Raise

Caution: If you suffer from lower back problems, a better exercise would be the calf press. With this exercise, your back has to support the weight being lifted. Additionally, your back needs to be straight and still at all times. If you round your back, this can cause a lower back injury.

1. Start by adjusting the padded lever to fit your height on the standing calf raise machine.

2. Place your shoulders under the pads and position your toes forward with your feet at shoulder-width apart. The balls of your feet should be on top of the calf block and your heels should be extending off the end.

3. Push the weight up by extending your knees until you're standing erect. Your knees should have a slight bend and never be fully locked.

4. Push through the balls of your feet to raise your heels while flexing your calves. There should be no bending in your knees at any time. Hold for a second before you begin to return back down.

5. Slowly lower your heels and the weight as you bend your ankles until you feel a stretch in your calves.

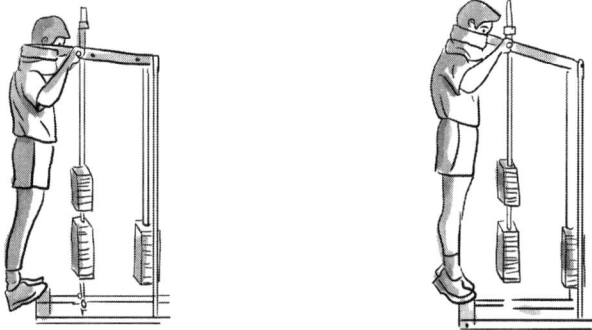

Seated Calf Press Machine

1. Sit on the machine and place your toes on the lower portion of the platform provided with the heels extending off.

2. Lift your heels up by pushing off your toes.

3. Release the safety bar.

4. Allow your heel to return towards the floor slowly, and then push through your toes to lift your heels again. Repeat until the set is complete.

5. Return the weight and safety bar to their starting positions.

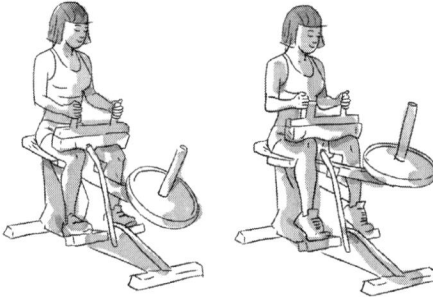

Shoulder Workouts

Glute Hamstring Extension

1. Set up with the knees either directly on or slightly behind the pad, with the feet firmly on the platform and the back of the calves pressed lightly against the upper ankle hook.

2. Begin with the torso perpendicular to the floor.

3. Next, squeeze the hamstrings, glutes, and abs, and lower under control until the torso is parallel to the floor.

4. From there, return to the starting position by pushing the toes into the foot plate (which activates the gastrocnemius) and pulling up with the hamstrings. Be sure to keep the glutes contracted.

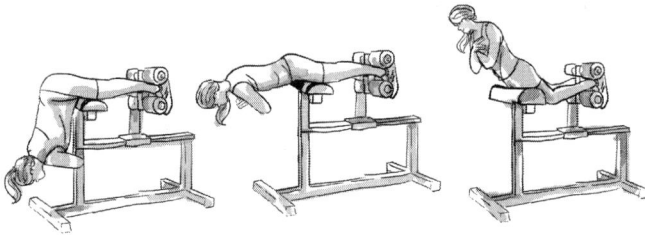

Barbell Raise

1. Stand upright with your feet shoulder-width apart. Grasp the barbell with an overhand grip that is slightly less than shoulder-width apart. The bar should be in front of your thighs with your arms extended and your palms facing your body.

2. Use the sides of your shoulders to lift the bar up towards your chest and drive your elbows up and to the side. Keep the bar close to your body as you raise it.

3. While keeping your elbows flared out, continue to lift the bar until it's at your upper chest level. Keep your torso stationary and pause for a second at the top of the movement.

4. Slowly lower the bar back to the starting position.

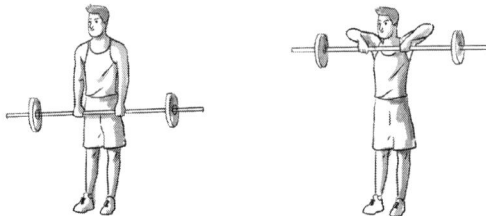

Bent Over Rear Delt Raise

1. Hold a dumbbell in each hand.

2. Bend at the hip with the butt back as far as possible.

3. Keep the back straight in order to pick up the dumbbells. The palms of your hands should be facing each other as you hold the dumbbells. This will be your starting position.

4. Keeping your torso forward and stationary and the arms slightly bent at the elbows, lift the dumbbells straight to the side until both arms are parallel to the floor. (Note: Avoid swinging the torso or bringing the arms back as opposed to the side.)

5. After a one second contraction at the top, slowly lower the dumbbells back to the starting position.

   Variation: This exercise can also be performed seated. Those with lower back problems are better off performing this seated variety.

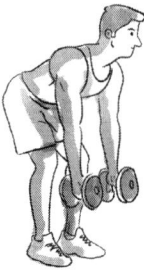

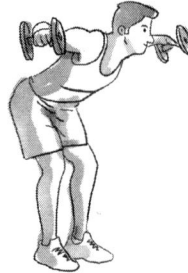

Shoulder Workouts

Front Dumbbell Raise

1. Stand upright with your feet hip-width apart. Grasp one dumbbell with each hand so that your palms are facing inward and hands are against your thighs.

2. While keeping your torso stationary, lift the dumbbells in front of you with a straight arm or slightly bent elbow. Continue to raise the dumbbell until your arm is slightly above parallel to the ground or around shoulder-level.

3. Slowly lower the dumbbells back to the starting position.

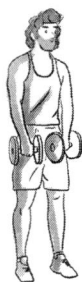

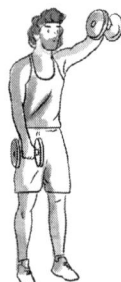

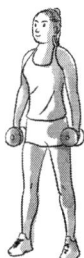

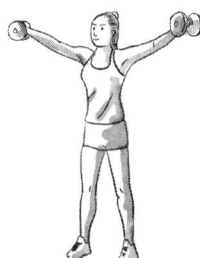

Lateral Dumbbell Raise

1. Stand upright with your feet shoulder-width apart and dumbbells aligned with your feet at arm's length. Make sure your palms are facing inward towards your sides.

2. Keep your torso stationary and raise the dumbbells to your side with a slight bend at your elbow. Lift your arms until they are slightly parallel to the ground, or around shoulder-level, and pause for a second at the top.

3. Slowly lower the dumbbells back to the starting position.

Reverse Fly

1. On the reverse fly machine (which sometimes doubles as a chest fly machine), adjust the handles so that they are fully facing the rear (closest together). Adjust the seat height to make the handles at your shoulder-level. Sit on the seat with your chest against the pad and grasp the handles with your palms facing inwards.

2. Pull your hands out to your sides and back as far as possible. This should make a semicircular motion where you should feel a stretch in your shoulders.

3. Pause at the back of the movement, and slowly return the weight to the starting position.

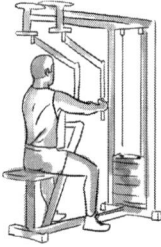

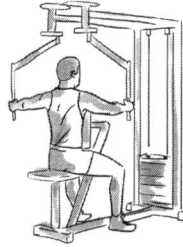

Shoulder Workouts

Shrugs

1. Stand upright or very slightly bent over with one dumbbell in each hand. Your palms should be facing your torso or each other and your arms should be fully extended by your sides.

2. Lift the dumbbells by raising your shoulders as high as possible towards your ears while keeping your arms fully extended. Hold the contraction at the top for at least half a second.

3. Lower the dumbbells back to the original position. Your shoulder should be the only part moving for this movement.

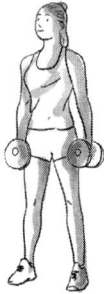

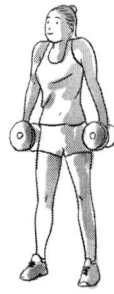

Reverse Dumbbell Fly

1. Grab a dumbbell in each hand with the palms facing each other (neutral grip). Bend your torso so that you're at a 90 degree angle, with your torso parallel to the floor.

2. Let your arms hang with the dumbbells in them.

3. Maintaining the slight bend of the elbows, move the weights out and away from each other (to the side) in an arc motion while. **Try to raise them as high as possible, aiming to squeeze your shoulder blades together.**

4. The arms should be elevated until they are parallel to the floor.

5. Feel the contraction and slowly lower the weights back down to the starting position.

6. Repeat for the recommended amount of repetitions.

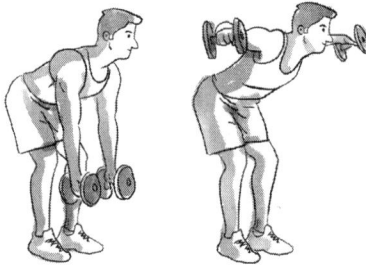

Tricep Workouts

Assisted Dip

1. Stand on the bottom step and grasp the handles half-way up the frame with an overhand grip.

2. Kneel on the pad while grasping the handles to test the pad pressure.

3. Adjust the upward pressure (more weight equals more assistance) on the pad to the point where you can do a set.

4. As you get stronger, decrease the upward support gradually.

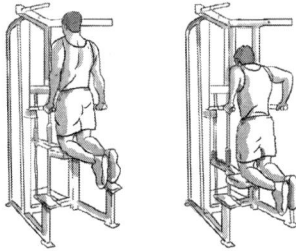

Diamond Push-Up

1. Start by lying on the floor face down with your hands closer than shoulder-width apart. Hold your torso up at arm's length.

2. Lower yourself until your chest almost touches the floor.

3. Using your triceps, press your upper body back up and squeeze your chest.

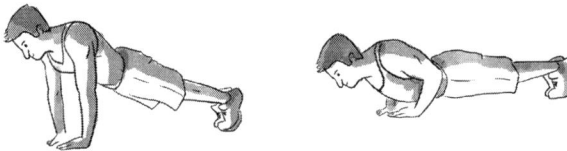

Tricep Workouts

Dip

1. Hold your body above the bars with your arms fully extended and nearly locked into the starting position.

2. Inhale and slowly lower yourself downward. Your torso should remain upright and your elbows should stay close to your body to help to better work your triceps. Lower yourself until a 90° angle is created between your upper arms and forearms.

3. Exhale and push your torso back up using your triceps (feeling a slight stretch in your shoulders) to bring your body back to the starting position.

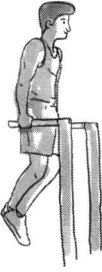

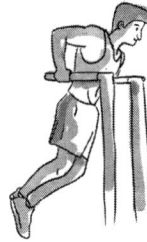

Tricep Workouts

Overhead Dumbbell Extension

1. Stand upright with a single dumbbell held by both hands. Your feet should be positioned about shoulder-width apart. Use both hands to lift the dumbbell over your head until both arms are fully extended.

2. To start, your palms are supporting the weight of the dumbbell with your thumbs wrapping around it. Your palms should be facing upward, maintaining an overlapped grip.

3. Keep your upper arms close to your head and perpendicular to the ground with your elbows by your ears. Lower the dumbbell in a semicircular motion behind your head so that your forearms touch (or almost touch) your biceps. Your forearms should be the only part moving.

4. Use your triceps to lower the dumbbell back to the starting position.

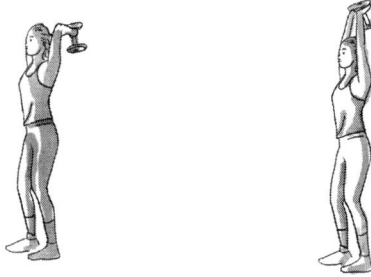

Rope Pulldown

1. Secure a rope attachment to the high pulley at its highest position. Stand in front of the pulley, hinge at your hips, and grab the rope with your palms facing each other.

2. Keep your elbows close to your torso, while using your triceps to pull the rope downwards toward the outside of your thighs. At the most contracted point of the motion, your arms should be fully extended and perpendicular to the ground. Your forearms should be the only part moving.

3. After reaching the contracted position, slowly bring the rope up to the starting point.

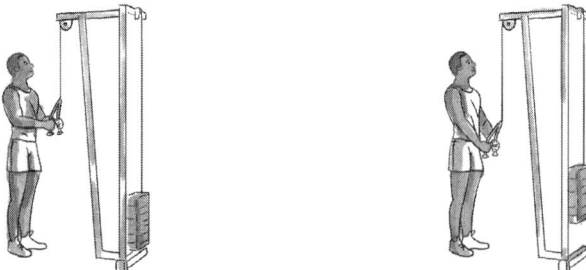

Tricep Workouts

Seated Dip w/ Machine

1. Sit securely in the dip machine and firmly grasp the handles.

2. Pin your elbows to your sides in order to maximize focus on your triceps. Make sure to keep your elbows bent at a 90° angle.

3. As you contract your triceps, fully extend your arms downward. Try to keep your arms slightly bent to create the most tension on your triceps.

4. Slowly let your arms return to the starting position.

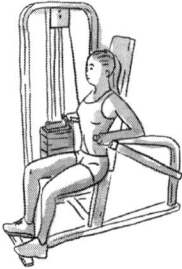

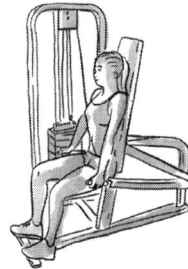

Skull Crusher

1. Lie back on a flat or slightly inclined bench. Using an overhand grip, grasp the innermost grips on the EZ bar. Hold it with your elbows tucked in and your arms perpendicular to the ground.

2. Keeping your upper arms stationary, lower the bar by unlocking your elbows to a flexed position. Pause once the bar is directly above your forehead.

3. Reverse the bar back to the starting position by extending your elbows while flexing your tricep.

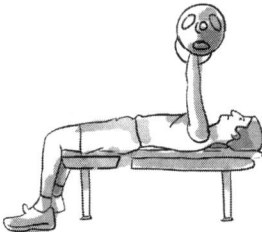

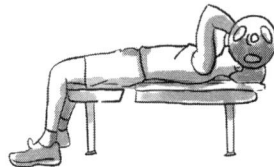

Tricep Workouts

Dumbbell Pullover

Caution: Always ensure that the dumbbell used for this exercise is secure.

1. Sit on a flat bench with one dumbbell resting on your thigh.

2. Lie back on the bench with your feet on the ground and your head hanging over the end. Grasp the dumbbell with both hands and hold it directly over your chest at arm's length.

3. Both of your palms should be pressing against the underside of the dumbbell.

4. While keeping your arms straight, lower the weight above and beyond your head until your upper arms are aligned with your torso. You should feel a stretch in your chest.

5. Lift the dumbbell back up and over your chest to the starting position.

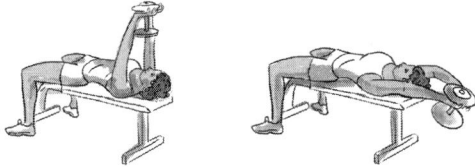

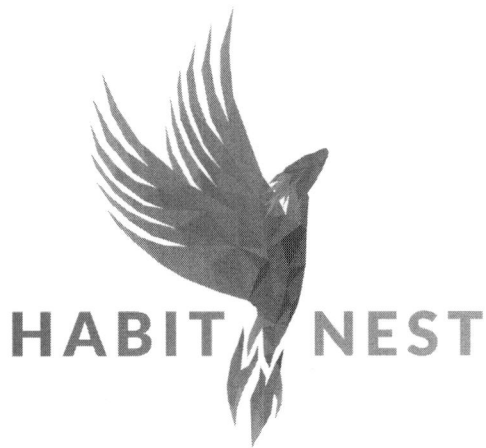

HABIT NEST

Your home for building healthy lifestyle habits.

HabitNest.com